Identifying and Understanding
the Narcissistic Personality

Identifying and Understanding the Narcissistic Personality

Elsa F. Ronningstam

OXFORD
UNIVERSITY PRESS

2005

OXFORD
UNIVERSITY PRESS

Oxford University Press, Inc., publishes works that further
Oxford University's objective of excellence
in research, scholarship, and education.

Oxford   New York
Auckland   Cape Town   Dar es Salaam   Hong Kong   Karachi
Kuala Lumpur   Madrid   Melbourne   Mexico City   Nairobi
New Delhi   Shanghai   Taipei   Toronto

With offices in
Argentina   Austria   Brazil   Chile   Czech Republic   France   Greece
Guatemala   Hungary   Italy   Japan   Poland   Portugal   Singapore
South Korea   Switzerland   Thailand   Turkey   Ukraine   Vietnam

Published by Oxford University Press, Inc.
198 Madison Avenue, New York, New York 10016

www.oup.com

Oxford is a registered trademark of Oxford University Press

Library of Congress Cataloging-in-Publication Data
Ronningstam, Elsa.
Identifying and understanding the narcissistic personality /
Elsa F. Ronningstam.
  p. cm.
Includes bibliographical references and index.
ISBN-13 978-0-19-514873-2
ISBN 0-19-514873-8
1. Narcissism. I. Title.
RC553.N36R66 2005
616.85'854—dc22   2004017142

9 8 7 6 5 4 3 2 1

Printed in the United States of America
on acid-free paper

To the memory of my mother,
Frideborg Rönnberg Karlsson

Credits

Chapter 1 is partly adapted from Ronningstam, E. (2005). Narcissistic personality disorder: A review. In M. Maj, H. Akiskal, J. Mezzich, & A. Okasha (Eds.), *The World Psychiatric Association series: Volume 8. Evidence & experiences in psychiatry: Personality disorders* (pp. 281–333). Chichester: John Wiley & Sons.

Chapter 2 is partly adapted from Ronningstam, E. (2003). Foreword. In E. Ronningstam (Ed.), *Disorders of narcissism: Diagnostic, clinical, and empirical implications* (Jpn. ed., pp. 3–7). Washington, DC: American Psychiatric Press and John Scott & Company. (Originally published 1998).

Chapter 4 is partly adapted from Ronningstam, E. (2005). Narcissistic personality disorder: A review. In M. Maj, H. Akiskal, J. Mezzich, & A. Okasha (Eds.), *The World Psychiatric Association series: Vol. 8. Evidence & experiences in psychiatry: Personality disorders* (pp. 281–333). Chichester: John Wiley & Sons.

Chapter 5 is partly adapted from Ronningstam, E. (1996). Pathological narcissism and narcissistic personality disorder in Axis I disorders. *Harvard Review of Psychiatry, 3*, 326–340; and Ronningstam, E. (2005). Narcissistic personality disorder: A review. In M. Maj, H. Akiskal, J. Mezzich, & A. Okasha (Eds.), *The World Psychiatric Association series, Vol. 8: Evidence & experiences in psychiatry: Personality disorders* (pp. 281–333). Chichester: John Wiley & Sons.

Chapter 6 is partly adapted from Ronningstam, E., & D. Anick. (2000). The interrupted career group—a preliminary report. *Harvard Review of Psychiatry, 9*, 234–243.

Chapter 7 is partly adapted from Ronningstam, E., & J. Maltsberger. (1998). Pathological narcissism and sudden suicide-related collapse. *Suicide and Life-Threatening Behavior, 28*(3), 261–271; and Ronningstam, E. (2000). Suicidal behavior in narcissistic patients. In *Directions in clinical and counseling psychology* (Vol. 10, Lesson 7, pp. 73–82). New York: Hatherleigh Company.

Chapter 8 is adapted from Ronningstam, E. (In press). Changes in narcissistic psychopathology—the influence of corrective and corrosive life-events. In O. Kernberg & H. Hartman (Eds.), *Narzisstische Persönlichkeitsstörnungen*. Stuttgart: Schattauer Verlag.

Introduction

Over the past century numerous studies on narcissism and narcissistic disorders have added to our present understanding of these conditions. Although there is by now a general agreement about the dynamics and features of pathological narcissism and narcissistic personality disorder (abbreviated NPD throughout this volume), there are still different and contradictory opinions about conceptualization and clinical descriptions of these conditions. The complex nature of pathological narcissism and the challenges involved in treating narcissistic patients have been major contributing factors. The official diagnostic system, Axis II of *The Diagnostic and Statistical Manual of Mental Disorders* (4th ed. and 4th ed. text revision; American Psychiatric Association, 1994, 2000; abbreviated *DSM-IV* throughout this volume), has presented some limitations in capturing personality pathology and reflecting the clinicians' usage of personality disorder diagnosis. This has been particularly consequential for diagnosing patients with narcissistic disorders. People with pathological narcissism that range beyond the *DSM-IV* criteria set, or people who have less extensive or less overt narcissistic disorders or who may show (even severe) pathological narcissism that is more specifically situational or contextually determined (e.g., expressed only within the marriage or in the workplace), tend to be overlooked and not correctly identified. In addition, the definitions and dynamic meaning and expressions of several of the characteristics for pathological narcissism are vague, and the vicissitudes in interpersonal interactions, self-esteem fluctuations, and affect dysregulation have until recently remained a relatively unexplored area.

This book is an attempt to translate studies of narcissism, that is, of specific narcissistic features and NPD, into the daily clinical practice of diagnosing and understanding people with disordered narcissism. In other words, this book represents an attempt to bridge the gaps between psychoanalytic, psychological, and psychiatric studies and to provide a first integrated clinical and empirical guideline to assist clinicians in their work with narcissistic patients. The long tradition of psychoanalytic observations and theory building on individual psychopathology, the academic psychological laboratory ratings of human functioning within a relatively normal range, and the psychiatric and psychosocial research efforts to find evidence of generalized and prototypical features have all interfaced in the studies of narcissism. The diversity and tension between these different methods offer a creative and very promising opportunity to enhance our knowledge and understanding. They also enable a choice between methods of observation and verification that can be better adjusted to the complex nature of narcissism and to individual variations.

This volume refers to narcissism as a dimension ranging from healthy and normal to pathological and to the long-term enduring arrogant NPD. It also positions pathological narcissism in a context ranging from "shy" NPD to psychopathic NPD. Based on an overview of available clinical and empirical studies, I have outlined some of the major characteristics of narcissistic self-esteem regulation, affect regulation, and interpersonal relativeness. Regulations of shame and aggression as well as specific narcissistic superego functioning are also addressed.

This book was written in the aftermath of the intense worldwide discussions on NPD during the 1970s and 1980s. The groundbreaking psychoanalytic contributions of Heinz Kohut and Otto Kernberg in the end of the 1960s inspired new conceptualizations of pathological narcissism. In addition, new theoretical and clinical approaches have developed for studying and treating narcissistic disorders that reflect far beyond the psychoanalytic realm. The introduction of NPD in Axis II of the *DSM* in 1980 opened the door for empirical studies of pathological narcissism and NPD as part of cluster B personality disorders. Since then, the academic nonclinical psychological studies on narcissism have proven to be increasingly valuable, providing important and clinically relevant information on the relations among narcissism, self-esteem, and affect dysregulation. Furthermore, studies of narcissism have moved into applied areas such as the workplace and suicidology, and several recent psychoanalytic contributions have suggested new and more efficient treatment approaches that are adjusted to the specific nature of disordered narcissism.

As its title indicates, this book is mainly devoted to identifying and understanding narcissism, both in its healthy and in its pathological forms. I have left a thorough discussion of treatment for narcissistic disorders for a future volume, but address it briefly in chapter 7 in a section on treatment of suicidality in narcissistic patients and in chapter 8 on changes in pathological narcissism. The vast developments in current integrative treatment modalities, especially in the field of personality disorders, as well as new treatment developments in psychoanalysis and psychoanalytic psychotherapy, are beyond the scope of this volume.

The importance of a historical context when defining the presence and outlining the future was pointed out by the Danish philosopher Kierkegaard, who stated that "life must be lived forward but understood backward." In other words, history is to be the guide for the future, and I believe that is particularly true for studies of narcissism. The rich and complex historical accounts on narcissism are described in chapter 1, "From Myth to Personality Disorder."

The purpose of chapter 2, "A Normal Asset With Cultural Differences," is to provide a basis for understanding the complex vicissitudes of healthy and pathological narcissism. Most of the characteristics that are considered core symptoms of pathological narcissism do indeed have their normal, healthy counterpart, for example, the personal sense of rights and expectations in normal entitlement, as compared to the pathological grandiose self-righteousness with unreasonable expectations in narcissistic entitlement, and the motivational role of grandiose fantasies in normal narcissism versus the defensive or self-enhancing function of pathological grandiose fantasies. In my work with people with narcissistic disorders, I have found it increasingly important to identify and highlight healthy narcissistic strivings, especially as they intertwine with pathological self-criticism, shame, and aggression.

Chapter 3, "The Origins and the Scope," discusses the heritability and the early development that may promote pathological narcissistic functioning, and specific childhood roles and experiences that contribute to narcissistic character development. Available data on prevalence, age, and gender differences of NPD are also included.

In chapter 4, "Identifying Pathological Narcissism," each characteristic is discussed in depth, and observations from both psychoanalytic and empirical studies are integrated into a dynamic description of each characteristic. The purpose is to identify the core features and to capture the range and variations of narcissistic pathology. This chapter proposes a set of identifying diagnostic criteria for NPD and differentiating criteria for both shy and psychopathic NPD.

The co-occurrence of pathological narcissism and NPD in other personality disorders and major mental disorders is discussed in the chapter 5, "Differentiating Pathological Narcissism." I have paid specific attention to the narcissistic meaning and function of co-occurring symptoms and dynamics of other disorders.

Chapters 6 and 7 attempt to apply the discussions in preceding chapters to two major contexts in which pathological narcissism recently has proven to be particularly consequential: the workplace, and suicidality. Narcissism in the workplace can represent both valuable leadership qualities or outstanding individual performance, and unproductive self-esteem fluctuations or organizational exploitation, as discussed in chapter 6, "Asset or Disruption?" The role of pathological narcissism in suicide has been more acknowledged since recent studies have shown that suicidal behaviors occur even when people do not feel depressed, unhappy, hopelessness, or guilty. In narcissistic patients, the idea of suicide can raise the self-esteem; contribute to a sense of superiority, mastery, and control; and protect against threats and injuries. In chapter 7, "My Way or No Way," diagnosis and treatment of narcissistically charged suicidal ideations and behavior are discussed.

Finally, chapter 8, "Correction or Corrosion," addresses changes in pathological narcissism. People with narcissistic personalities have been considered especially resistant to change through treatment. Nevertheless, studies have shown that narcissistic people are specifically susceptible to life experiences than can both decrease and increase pathological narcissism.

Acknowledgments

This book is the result of more than 20 years of studies of narcissism both in my roles as a researcher, author, and editor and in my role as a clinician and candidate in psychoanalytic training.

I first thank my patients, who have provided me with the most detailed knowledge. Their courage and persistence in conveying their challenging inner experiences and accepting my efforts to explore, understand, and treat them have been invaluable. I also thank my students and my clinical and research supervisees, who likewise have shared with me their experiences and provided guiding feedback.

Many people—mentors, teachers and supervisors, research and clinical colleagues, and peers—have over the years contributed in various ways, some more directly, others indirectly, to my work on narcissism. I have specifically learned from John Gunderson, John Maltsberger, AnaMaria Rizzuto, Ralf Beaumonth, David Berkowitch, and Lewis Kirshner, and I thank them for outstanding mentorship and supervision. Over the years I have also learned and received valuable support and inspiration from Otto Kernberg, Paulina Kernberg, and Arnold Cooper. Theodor Millon, Erik Simonsen, and Per Vaglum have all encouraged and supported my work over the past 15 years, especially through our collaboration in the International Society for the Studies of Personality Disorder. I also thank my colleagues at McLean Hospital—the Personality Disorder Program and the Borderline Center—as well as at Two Brattle Center in Cambridge and in the Boston Suicide Study Group, for their devoted clinical collaboration and inspiring discussions. These affiliations have been invaluable sources of constructive feedback and support of my professional growth.

My first mentor, Professor C.-O. Jonsson, Department of Psychology, University of Stockholm, deserves special thanks for his faithful and persistent support and encouragement during my formative training years. Likewise, I am also grateful to my supervisors Clarence Crafford and Robert Rössel, psychoanalysts in Stockholm, who inspired and encouraged my psychoanalytic studies of borderline and narcissistic patients. I will always remember my colleagues at the former Department of Psychology at Beckomberga Hospital in Stockholm, who first introduced me to the inspiring studies on narcissism.

In the process of writing this book, Dr. Igor Weinberg provided valuable comments and advice. I give special thanks to my editorial secretary and advisor Marietta Pritchard for her thorough and helpful editorial advice. Finally, for his patience, inspiration, and warm encouraging support, I thank my husband, Philip.

Contents

1. From Myth to Personality Disorder   3

2. A Normal Asset With Cultural Differences   31

3. The Origins and Scope of Narcissistic
   Personality Disorder   49

4. Identifying Pathological Narcissism   69

5. Differentiating Pathological Narcissism   113

6. Asset or Disruption? Narcissism in the Workplace   135

7. My Way or No Way! Narcissism and Suicide   159

8. Correction or Corrosion? Changes
   in Pathological Narcissism   181

Epilogue   197

Appendix   201

References   203

Index   233

Identifying and Understanding
the Narcissistic Personality

1

From Myth to Personality Disorder

The Antecedents

Paradoxically, the Narcissus myth by Ovid (Melville, 1986, pp. 61–66), which in our time has come to represent self-love or self-reflection, actually described the tragic inability to love at all (Winge, 1967). It is the story of a beautiful young man, son of the river nymph Liriope and the river god Cephisus, whose destiny—to die young if he gets to know himself—had been early prophesied. Because of his cold, hard pride, Narcissus could not be touched by the many young boys and girls who loved him, not even by Echo, whose "heart was fired" by the sight of him. When Narcissus fell in love with the image in the pool, he mistakenly took it for a real body and did not understand that it was a reflection of his own body. In other words, Narcissus could not conceive that he was in love with his own reflection; he was caught in an illusion. All efforts to converse with the unreachable image in the spring left Narcissus disheartened and filled with despair. Finally he realized: "I am he! Oh, now I know for sure the image is my own; it's for myself I burn with love; I fan the flames I feel" (Melville, 1986, pp. 64–65). Heartbroken, he wished he could separate himself from his own body so that the image he loved would go away. He then sensed that death was the only solution as "now we two—one soul—one death will die" (p. 65). He faded away, and when the nymphs came to bury his body, they found a flower at its place.

How the narcissus myth came to represent self-love or self-admiration is unclear, but in art and literature during the medieval and early Renaissance eras the theme was used to illustrate the dangerous sinfulness and deadly punishment attached to excessive self-preoccupation and self-adulation. Calderon de la Barca in the seventeenth century was the first to transform the classic description of Narcissus into a modern interactive stage play about the young man in *Eco y Narciso* (*Echo and Narcissus*; de la Barca, 1661/1976). Calderon moved away from moral condemnation of excessive self-love and created a dynamic outline of Narcissus (Gran, 1976). He explained Narcissus's love of his own reflection not as self-love but as a flight, a consequence of incompatible conflicts and desires in a young man, still attached to his domineering and protecting mother, confused by Echo's alternation between seductive invitation and mute rejection, and torn between warnings and ill-fated male advice. In other words, Calderon de la Barca introduced an interpersonal perspective to the Narcissus myth, and he was the avant-garde to what later was defined as narcissistic affect dysregulation, as he staged Narcissus's struggle with sudden intense and overwhelming sexual feelings, inner pride, and shame and confusion. With no natural outlet for his strong feelings, Narcissus turned to himself and his image in the spring, and died.

Another Spanish writer, Juan Valera, who was closer to modern thinking on narcissism as autoerotic self-love or admiration, described in his novel *Genio y Figura* (1897) the heroine Rafaela. She confessed that when looking in the mirror she was filled with love and admiration for herself, and she imitated Narcissus and kissed her own beautiful image on the surface of the mirror. But contrary to Narcissus, Rafaela was fully aware of the separateness of her own physical body and self from the image of her body she perceived in the mirror. She was also fully capable of experiencing pleasure. Valera's novel inspired both Havelock Ellis and J. Sadger in their psychological and psychoanalytic accounts of narcissism and female autoerotism (Ellis, 1928, pp. 352, 355).

The Narcissus theme has also inspired numerous artists. One of the earliest known attempts to portray Narcissus appears in a wall painting in Pompeii. During the Renaissance, several artists chose Narcissus to illustrate self-love, self-admiration, and the contemplation of one's own image. Caravaggio's *Narcissus* and Velasquez's and Titan's portraits of Venus are well-known examples. It is notable that the young Narcissus was gradually replaced by images of women who represented the fatal sin of self-admiration and vanity. In many paintings, among others by Baldung (sixteenth century), attractive women looking at themselves in the mirror are threatened by figures representing Death. In the twentieth century, the theme became one of mirroring and preoccupation with appearance, self-recognition, and self-regard, as in Norman Rockwell's *Girl in the Mirror* and the etching titled *Adolescence* by the British artist Gerald Leslie Brockhurst. The themes of reflection and mirroring were specifically featured in an exhibition, "Mirror Image," at the National Gallery in London and further discussed in an accompanying book by J. Miller (1998).

Early Psychiatric and Psychoanalytic Development

Ellis (1898) introduced the phenomenon of narcissism to psychiatry in his psychological study of autoeroticism, in which he described the "Narcissus-like" tendency to absorb sexual feelings into self-admiration (p. 280). The following year, Paul Näcke (1899) was first to use the term "narcissism" in a study of sexual perversions. Freud first mentioned narcissism in a footnote added in 1910 to "Three Essays on the Theory of Sexuality" (Freud, 1905/1957), as a phase in the development of male homosexuality. In 1911 (Freud, 1911/1957) he referred to narcissism as the choice of self as a libidinal object, a normal stage of autoerotism in the early libidinal development. The concept was by then acknowledged among psychoanalysts, and in subsequent accounts narcissism was considered both a part of normal development and human functioning and a type of deviation or perversion.

In the first psychoanalytic paper on narcissism, Rank (1911) discussed the development of self-love, specifically expressed through a woman's dreams and her experience of being unable to love a man unless she first knows that he loves her. Freud, in his main paper on the subject, "On Narcissism" (1914/1957), and in his later comments (1915/1957, 1917/1957), outlined definitions of primary and secondary narcissism, identified narcissistic object choice, and connected narcissism to the development of the ego-ideal and to self-preservation and self-regard as the "libidinal complement of egoism." Another important observation of much relevance for the contemporary discussion of narcissism concerned the relationship between narcissism and inferiority. Freud suggested that the impoverishment of the ego due to the withdrawal of libidinal cathexis (investment of sexual drive energy) contributed to feelings of inferiority. In addition, he identified the role of narcissism in sleep and dreams and in the process of falling in love. Sadger (1910), another European psychoanalyst, viewed narcissism as a normal phenomenon, an overvaluation of oneself seen in children and in a certain degree of self-love among adults, but its fixations and extreme manifestations, such as the overvaluation of one's own body, he considered to be pathological. He differentiated between normal egoism and narcissism, and suggested that friendship is an extended form of narcissism. The first American discussion on narcissism took place in 1915 in New York, at the sixth annual meeting of the American Psychopathological Association (1915). The program included a paper by J. S. Van Teslaar titled "Narcissism."

The connection between narcissism and self-esteem regulation, first alluded to by Freud in his discussion of self-regard and the development of the ego-ideal (1914/1957), was further developed by Horney (1939), who differentiated healthy self-esteem from pathological unrealistic self-inflation, a substitute for an undermined self-esteem. Anne Reich (1960) added considerably to the understanding of pathological self-esteem regulation, which, in her opinion, serves to maintain grandiosity and undo feelings of inadequacy and insufficiency. She described the strategy of compensatory narcissistic self-inflation, which fails and results in hypochondriac anxiety and depression. Excessive inner aggression and inordinate self-consciousness leading to dependency on outside approval contribute to these regulation failures. Kohut (1971) identified defects in self-esteem regulation as one of the core disturbances in narcissistic personality disorder (NPD), and Goldberg (1973) proposed a separate diagnostic category of acute narcissistic injury to one's self-esteem that may manifest itself as depression but should be differentiated and treated differently from general depressive reactions or disorder.

In the first account on treatment of narcissistic disorder, Wälder (1925) outlined the difference between narcissism and psychosis, an essential distinction, as it was clear by then that the transference technique was not applicable either for narcissistic fixations or for psychosis. He discussed a technique focusing on "sublimation of narcissism," changing the narcissistic attachment to the objects within the subject's own ego, and "the mode of union of narcissism with these objects" (p. 273). At the Ninth International Psychoanalytic Congress, Clark (1926) proposed another therapeutic technique for narcissistic patients, "the fantasy method of analyzing narcissistic neurosis." By introducing a "mild self-hypnosis," not unlike daydreaming, a "disorganization of consciousness" occurred that could promote the development of a narcissistic transference. This process aimed at uncovering the narcissistic individual's primary personality and accessing memories of early mother–child interactions. The individual could then be helped to gain the ability to sublimate and to gain insight into disabling narcissistic patterns, as well as to maintain the degree of narcissism that could be beneficial for overall well-being.

Narcissistic Personalities

Long before the introduction of the diagnosis of NPD in the late 1960s, numerous authors have described in great detail the complexity of this personality functioning. Few personalities have lent themselves to the imagination of subtypes and variations as well as has the narcissistic personality, and few have been observed and documented with such fascination, puzzlement, and awe. The accounts have shown unusual diversity and even opposing and contradicting features, both within the field of literature and within psychiatry/psychoanalysis.

In a remarkable, thoughtful, observant, and still most timely report, Jones (1913/1951) described the character traits of people with a "God complex." He suggested that the excessive narcissism and exhibitionism involved in such a fantasy of being God or godlike and the accompanying admiration of one's own power and qualities were manifested in a range of character traits. Contrary to later accounts of narcissistic personalities, Jones highlighted self-modesty, self-effacement, aloofness, and inaccessibility as the main features of this narcissistic personality. Narcissistic persons are surrounded by a cloud of mystery; they are unsociable and protective of their privacy. Jones distinguished between two major types: those whose qualities indeed are valuable, adaptable, and truly godlike and those whose unrealistic self-evaluation and difficulties in adjusting to social life leave them dissatisfied and outside.

Wälder (1925) discussed the intellectual functioning of the "narcissistic scientist," a person with a superior attitude and who, although fully able to understand others intellectually, still is indifferent to them. He described a mathematician who was preoccupied with concepts and tended to prize the knowledge itself before its application. The main striving of this character was to fit theories into a logical systematic structure that enabled him to build constructs and make reductions as needed, in other words, a pursuit "to create a world for oneself." When this failed, a state of dissociation occurred as if he had become two people inside. Indifference was the best protection against disappointment. Because of his profession, this man could withdraw from relationships and still stay connected with reality, avoiding psychotic regression by engaging in intellectual productivity.

After these earliest thoughtful and subtle accounts, the descriptions of narcissistic personalities became more influenced by the connection between narcissism and aggression. Freud (1931/1957) introduced the "narcissistic libidinal type": "The subject's main interest is directed to self-preservation; he is independent and not open to intimidation. His ego has a large amount of aggressiveness at its disposal, which also manifests itself in readiness for activity. In his erotic life loving is preferred above being loved. People belonging to this type impress others as being 'personalities'; they are especially suited to act as a support for others, to take on the role of leaders and to give a fresh stimulus to cultural development or to damage the established state of affairs." (p. 218). W. Reich (1933/1949) followed this view and proposed the phallic-narcissistic character, a self-confident, arrogant, vigorous, and impressive individual, an athletic type—hard and sharp with masculine features. These individuals are haughty, cold, reserved, or aggressive with disguised sadistic traits in relation to others. They resent subordination and readily achieve leading positions. When hurt, they react with cold reserve, deep depression, or intense aggression. Their narcissism is expressed in an exaggerated display of self-confidence, dignity, and superiority. They are often considered highly desirable as sexual partners because of their masculine traits, despite the fact that they usually show contempt for the female sex. Sexuality serves less as a vehicle of love than as one of aggression and conquest. Less frequent in women, Reich believed that the phallic-narcissistic character could develop either into a "creative genius or into a large scale criminal" (p. 206) depending upon capacity for genital gratification and opportunities for sublimation. He also noted that these characters could have the opposite features, that is, passive tendencies of daydreaming and addiction. These seminal characterizations of narcissistic personalities, although modified, still influence our present idea of NPD.

What followed after Freud and Reich was a series of clinical accounts of narcissistic characters that highlighted a broad range of characteristics, all captured under the umbrella concept of narcissistic character functioning. The focus was on achievements, grandiosity, and ambition. These influential descriptions further highlighted the diversity and complexity of the phenomenology of narcissistic personalities.

A "Nobel Prize complex" can, according to Tartakoff (1966), be found in some people who entertain ambitious goals. They are intellectually and artistically gifted, and admirable, and guided either by an active fantasy of being the powerful one (destined) or by a passive fantasy of being the special one (chosen). However, their achievements become overshadowed by their preoccupation with acclaim, an attitude of "all or nothing," or "dreams of glory," of attaining a position of extraordinary power or worldwide recognition. These people are dependent upon the evidence of their success, and they can become hypersensitive to the lack of such evidence. Loss of significant persons in their life can reveal their dependency. They either avoid or just lack the corrective experiences of facing their own limitations. Disappointments and failure may force these people to seek treatment in hope of the magical cure.

The "Don Juan of achievements" is a paradoxical phenomenon in narcissistic people, described by Fenichel (1945) as a driven wish for success that can undo previous failures and guilt but still leave the person without inner satisfaction. He described an ambitious man who, despite his significant external achievement and success, struggled with chronic dissatisfaction, feeling he could never satisfy his wish to become a great man. It seemed as if he was driven by the need for achievement to undo an inner sense of remaining like a child. In his relations to women, he felt chronic dissatisfaction, and his marriage was characterized by childish dependency, revenge, rage, unfaithfulness, and lack of consideration.

The "Icarus complex" was identified by Murray (1955) in a phallic-narcissistic character usually found among young people who are fixated on Icarian pursuits of unattainable goals. These characters have "peak and fall" experiences as they oscillate between periods of intense achievements or energetic, ecstatic activities characterized by "effortless mastery, and unconditioned admiration, and affection," and flat periods of dissatisfaction, emptiness, depression, boredom, and inability to find gratifying involvement (Weinberger & Muller, 1974, p. 581).

Volkan's (1979) narcissistic personality is enclosed in a fantasy of self-sufficiency, the "glass bubble fantasy," which functions like a protecting, invisible wall. This person's behavior is motivated by the idea of being unique and invulnerable, "impregnable in his solitary glory." The purpose of this "bubble" fantasy is to protect the cohesiveness of the person's grandiose self. Relations to others are characterized by a "nonrelativeness," a lack of emotional involvement. In psychoanalysis, the analyst becomes part of the patient's concept of his own grandiosity, like a confirmer.

Modell (1975, 1980, 1991) developed this notion further by suggesting that some people with NPD develop a defense against affects, like a "cocoon," or a "sphere within the sphere," or a "private self" that supports an illusion of self-sufficiency and protects against fear of intrusion from others. As analysands in psychoanalysis, they act as if they are talking to themselves, as if the analyst is not there. Nevertheless, Modell noticed that although these analysands do not communicate feelings and are seemingly not relating, they are still actively involved by seeking admiration and by maintaining the illusion of self-sufficiency and the idea that they do not need anything from others.

In addition, there are three recent contributions to the line of descriptions of narcissistic personalities. Inspired foremost by Jones (1913/1951), Akhtar (1989, 1997) outlined the "shy narcissistic personality" with more covert features of pathological narcissism. This type of narcissist also has grandiose fantasies, a sense of uniqueness, and a need for praise and recognition, but in contrast to the overt grandiose type, the shy narcissists hide their grandiose beliefs and aspirations, and appear modest and seemingly uninterested in social success. They have intact or even high moral standards. They are often aware of their inability to empathize, and they can actually be helpful and are able to feel grateful and even feel concern for others. Their impaired capacity for deep relations can be either hidden or apparent, but their yearnings for social contact, acceptance, and recognition are suppressed. They also feel shame when their grandiose ambitions are revealed and anxious when their exhibitionistic needs are exposed.

Following the idea of a personality with less visible narcissistic characteristics, Masterson (1993) introduced the "closet narcissist." Instead of developing a grandiose sense of self and their own sense of omnipotence, the closet narcissists choose to connect to special people whom they idealize and consider omnipotent. According to Masterson, they regulate their own grandiosity by "basking in the glow" (p. 21) of a special someone, hiding their own deep sense of inadequacy and deflation. Insufficient capacity to self-activate and maintain defenses makes the closet narcissist prone to humiliation and shame. In psychotherapy, such patients often idealize the therapist and act compliant.

Cooper (1981) noted that "self-esteem takes on a pathological quality when an individual begins to derive satisfaction from mastery of his own humiliations" (p. 314). He introduced the "narcissistic-masochistic character" (Cooper, 1981, 1988, 1989, 1998), with both narcissistic and masochistic traits, who has made suffering ego-syntonic and part of his or her own identity. Such a person experiences a sense of mastery and control by getting "satisfaction from angry self-pitying feelings of being injured" (Cooper, 1998, p. 65), believing that if one can tolerate and even enjoy disappointment, humiliation, and pain, one is protected and no longer at risk for getting hurt. It is a way to protect or restore threatened self-esteem. These narcissistic people may appear either charming and ambitious or depressed and aggressive.

Narcissistic Personality Disorder

The origin of narcissistic personality disorder (NPD) as a diagnostic category is more difficult to establish. Terms such as narcissistic neurosis, schizophrenia, and psychosis have often been used interchangeably, reflecting the initial close interrelation between narcissism and these illnesses. The theory of narcissistic and autoerotic regression (Freud, 1911/ 1957, 1914/1957) explained schizophrenic symptoms as a libidinal withdrawal from the object world and regression to a narcissistic stage. In addition, the observation that the capacity to develop classical transference during psychoanalysis was absent in patients diagnosed with narcissistic neurosis (Freud, 1914/1957) further connected narcissism and psychosis or schizophrenia. In addition, narcissism was associated with paranoia and suicide. Not until the late 1960s were the terms "narcissistic personality structure," introduced by O. Kernberg (1967), and "narcissistic personality disorder," proposed by Kohut (1968), used to describe a long-term organized characterological functioning defined as a personality disorder. Based on radical reformulations of psychoanalytic theory and technique, both Kohut and Kernberg defined NPD in terms of a pathological self-structure, atypical transference development, and strategies for psychoanalytic treatment.

Kohut included NPD in his diagnostic spectrum of primary self-disorders. He differentiated between "narcissistic personality disorder," with hypochondria, depression, hypersensitivity, and lack of enthusiasm/zest, and "narcissistic behavior disorder," which, in addition, includes perverse, delinquent, and/or addictive behavior that can expose the individual to physical or social danger (Kohut & Wolff, 1978). Kohut (1977) introduced the concept of the "tragic man" (p. 238), an additional contribution to the description of narcissistic personalities, who suffered from repressed grandiosity and guiltless despair. This person knows and understands that his ambitions have not been realized and that his self-realization has not occurred. He has failed to attain his goals for self-expression and creativity. Morrison (1983) stated that shame is the major distinguishing affective experience of the tragic man, shame caused by "the failure to realize ambitions, to gain response from others, at the absence of ideals" (p. 367). Kohut (1977) also described the individual with the "the depleted self," suffering from empty depression due to "unmirrored ambitions" and the absence of ideals (p. 243). To summarize, people with Kohut's NPD have repressed grandiosity, low self-esteem, and hypochondriacal preoccupation and are prone to shame and embarrassment about needs to display themselves and their needs for other people.

Inspired by Klein and Rosenfeld, O. Kernberg (1967, 1975) outlined patients with NPD as having a pathological grandiose self with aggression, excessive self-absorption, and superior sense of grandiosity and uniqueness. This narcissistic person has serious problems in interpersonal relations, with superficial but also smooth and effective social adaptation, entitlement, and lack of empathy. Kernberg's narcissistic personality shows devaluation, contempt, and depreciation of others, is extremely envious and unable to receive from others, and has severe mood swings. Kernberg also highlighted the presence of superego pathology in people with this diagnosis, a less severe level with lack of integrated sense of values, and a more severe level with "malignant narcissism"—antisocial features, ego-syntonic aggression and sadism, and a general paranoid orientation. Narcissistic pathology can be found in political leaders, selfless ideologists, and social redeemers (O. Kernberg, 1990, p. 5). However, Kernberg also recognized some atypical features found in patients with NPD: They can be anxious and tense, be timid and insecure, have grandiose fantasies and daydreams, be sexually inhibited, and have a lack of ambitions.

The Narcissistic-Borderline Merge

O. Kernberg (1975) included both NPD and borderline personality disorder (BPD) under the same structural diagnostic umbrella of "borderline personality organization." This diagnostic neighbor positioning inspired efforts to find conceptual relations between NPD and BPD. Numerous reports during the 1970s and 1980s addressed "borderline-narcissistic" or "narcissistic-borderline" disorders, their shared features, and opposite but related functioning. Other reports outlined treatment strategies for both disorders. Hartocollis (1980) believed that NPD and BPD shared disordered affects and mood, that is, a sense of inappropriateness, depersonalization, anger, feelings of emptiness and boredom, and a sense of injustice (NPD) and alienation (BPD). Lichtenberg (1987) noted that both NPD and BPD patients have "disturbance in the experience of the self as a cohesive, integrated, whole person" (p. 134). Both struggle with self-expansion and self-deflation and accompanying rage. In addition, NPD patients are unable to balance grandiose and deflated self-experiences with more stable and developmentally advanced self-experiences; that is, they are unable to regulate self-esteem.

Other authors preferred to place and compare the disorders as opposites or on a continuum. Grothstein (1984a, 1984b) suggested that NPD and BPD represent complementary but different defensive responses to painful affects connected with their perceptions of object relations. While narcissistic personalities develop manic defenses against vulnerability and helplessness and tend to take control over valued objects in order to incorporate the object's power within themselves, borderline personalities tend to accept their vulnerability and helplessness and develop an approach-withdrawal pattern in relation to the needed object. Adler (1981) believed that NPD and BPD constitute a developmentally based continuum wherein NPD patients have greater stability in self–object relatedness and more capacity for aloneness than do BPD patients. During the course of psychotherapy, BPD patients go through a process of change from being unable to maintain self-cohesiveness and positive images and memories of significant others, to being mainly preoccupied with issues related to self-worth (p. 48). Similarly, NPD patients can regress to a level of less cohesiveness. Although O. Kernberg (1984) claimed that NPD and BPD are separable by the more integrated but still pathological grandiose self-concept found in NPD, he suggested that some NPD patients can function on an overt borderline level with ego weakness and accompanying signs of lack of anxiety tolerance and impulse control, absence of sublimatory capacities, primary process thinking, and proneness to develop transference psychosis.

These initial efforts to find a conceptual relationship between NPD and BPD have been refuted over the past decade as both empirical and clinical evidence of the nature of these disorders has strongly pointed to their separateness. The degree of self-cohesiveness, tolerance for aloneness, capacity for and patterns of object relatedness, and etiology seem to be the core areas where the most significant differences between NPD and BPD have been identified. This is further discussed in chapter 5, which addresses differentiating NPD from other disorders.

Narcissistic Personality Typologies

Attempts to organize the different types of narcissistic personalities into typological systems were proposed by Ben Bursten and Theodore Millon. Although less frequently referred to, these sets of typologies highlight both the diversity and continuity of functional levels and symptom formations in pathological narcissism.

Bursten's Typology   Anchored in psychoanalytic theory, Bursten (1973) identified four types of narcissistic personalities based on their different modes of narcissistic repair, degrees of self-object differentiation, and types of value system: the craving, paranoid, manipulative, and phallic-narcissistic types.

The *craving type* is a dependent and passive aggressive person without the capacity to rely and depend on anyone, desperately and demandingly clinging, prone to disappointment, needy and craving attention, in constant need of being fed. As one patient who came to represent this extremely needy, narcissistic personality said, "I am like a bird with wide open beak." Anger is expressed as pouting and sulking, and craving personalities expect others to know their needs without having to tell them (excessive needy entitlement).

The *paranoid type* is a hypersensitive, rigid, suspicious, jealous, envious, and argumentative person, radiating excessive self-importance, blaming others and ascribing evil motives to them. Such people develop a mood of skepticism, criticism, and suspicion, and their anger ranges from skepticism to jealous rage. They are not delusional and can actually be high functioning.

The *manipulative type* shows more subtle forms of contempt and devaluation. People of this type are deceptive and feel contempt and exhilaration when a deception succeeds. They keep up their appearance by being clever and tricky, competitive, and focused on proving their superiority by defeating other people.

The *phallic narcissistic* type struggles with the shame of being weak, which is compensated for by competitiveness, pseudo-masculinity, aggressive and arrogant attitudes and self-glorification.

Millon's Typology   This is the most sophisticated typology capturing the complexity of narcissism derived from Millon's (1981, 1996, 1998) bio-social learning model for personality disorders. Each of the narcissistic subtypes consists of clinical domains (expressive behavior, interpersonal conduct, cognitive style, self-image, object representations, regulatory mechanisms, morphologic organization, and mood/temperament) and is organized according to its level of severity:

- The *normal narcissistic type* is by nature a competitive and self-assured person who believes in him- or herself. Charming, clever, confident, and ambitious, such a person often becomes an effective and successful leader.
- The *unprincipled type*—the charlatan—is a fraudulent, exploitative, deceptive, and unscrupulous individual. Although people displaying this type of narcissism are usually successful in society and manage to keep their activities within the accepted norms, they can also be found in drug rehabilitation programs, jails, and prisons.
- The *amorous type*—the Don Juan or Casanova of our times—is erotic, exhibitionistic and seductive, aloof, charming, exploitative, and reluctant to become involved in deep, mutual intimate relations.
- The *compensatory type* has illusions of superiority and an image of high self-worth, but with an underlying emptiness, insecurity, and weakness. This type is sensitive to others' reactions and prone to feeling ashamed, anxious, and humiliated.
- The *elitist type*—the achiever—corresponds to W. Reich's "phallic narcissistic" personality type, with excessively inflated self-image. This individual is elitist, a "social climber," superior, admiration seeking, self-promoting, bragging, and empowered by social success.
- The *fanatic type* is a severely narcissistically wounded individual, usually with major paranoid tendencies who holds on to an illusion of omnipotence. These people are fighting the reality of their insignificance and lost value and are trying to reestablish their self-esteem through grandiose fantasies and self-reinforcement. When unable to gain recognition or support from others, they take on the role of a heroic or worshipped person with a grandiose mission. These people can be found among sect leaders, in mental hospitals if their delusions become sustained and extensive, or in prison, if their missions counteract those of society.

While Millon's system is theoretically and empirically well anchored and captures an interesting and relevant range of diverse narcissistic pathology, it has proven most useful for research. Bursten's system is well-anchored in psychoanalytic theory and clinically meaningful because it identifies narcissistic types in terms of degrees of separation–individuation and value systems. However, it encompasses a limited although significant range of narcissistic character pathology.

Contemporary Perspectives and Controversies

Few disorders have as many theoretical and clinical antecedents as NPD. Although there is substantial agreement about some of its basic diagnostic features and etiology, a number of disagreements still remain. Contemporary psychoanalytic formulations diverge concerning the origin of the pathological grandiose self, primarily in their views about the role of aggression and envy and of primitive shame in early self development. They also disagree on the focus and technique of treatment of narcissistic people. The question of stability or cohesion of the pathological grandiose self and even the overt characteristics of narcissistic patients are subject to dispute. Biosocial learning theory has stimulated worldwide empirical research on NPD, and the diagnostic Millon Clinical Multiaxial Inventory (MCMI; Millon, Davis, & Millon, 1996) has been translated into nearly twenty languages and contributed to an international validation of this diagnostic category within both psychiatry and psychology. This theoretical perspective highlights environmental and parental influences on the development of an inflated self that is characterized by egotism, self-sufficiency, and learned entitled and exploitative behavior. A cognitive model for understanding NPD has instigated new treatment approaches outside the psychoanalytic realm. The most recent contribution is an empirical social-psychological model for self-regulation in narcissistic people (Morf & Rhodewalt, 2001; Rhodewalt & Sorrow, 2003). Although developed within the field of academic research, this model has proven to be specifically relevant for defining self-esteem regulation and certain narcissistic functioning.

The Psychoanalytic Perspective

Several psychoanalytic schools have made important contributions to the contemporary conceptualizations of pathological narcissism and narcissistic disorders, especially the British Society (Balint, 1959; Fairbairn, 1952; Hartman, 1964; Jacobson, 1964; M. Klein, 1957; Winnicott, 1953, 1965;), but also French psychoanalysis (Chasseguet-Smirgel, 1985; Grundberger, 1971; McDougall, 1985) and the Hungarian school (Ferenczi, 1913/1980). It is beyond the scope of this book to review the influence of the different psychoanalytic schools and their impact on the evolving understanding of narcissism. In addition, many detailed and unique psychoanalytic accounts of narcissism have influenced discussions throughout the years and added knowledge about the complexity of narcissistic personality functioning. I mention just a few of them here. In Germany, Henseler (1991) studied narcissism in terms of self-worth and reactions to narcissistic injuries, specifically the narcissistic catastrophe associated with suicidal behavior (see chapter 7). The work of Rosenfeld (1964, 1971) is relevant for understanding the intolerance of dependency and the role of envy in narcissistic people. He suggested that dependency makes the narcissistic person feel vulnerable to pain and separation. Good qualities in other people evoke a sense of humiliation and inferiority, and feelings of envy are warded off by devaluing or avoiding such people or by trying to destroy whatever good comes from them in order to protect self-esteem and maintain superiority.

Other significant individual contributions were made by Rothstein (1980), who connected narcissism with the striving for perfection and the defensive function of entitlement (see chapter 4 this volume), and Modell (1965, 1975, 1980), who explored specific features in narcissistic affect regulation, the non-communication of affects and striving for self-sufficiency, lack of empathy, and compromised entitlement (see chapter 4 this volume). Bach (1975, 1977b, 1985) was the first to describe the cognitive functioning of narcissistic people and their unusual way of using language for manipulative purposes to regulate self-esteem. He also described internal experiences and split off hyper- and hypoaroused states of the self with accompanying mood variations and shifts ranging from being in control and feeling omnipotent to having lost control and feeling helplessness, and from feeling elated and grandiose to experiencing inferiority and shame-dominant depression. While these shifts and oscillations usually represent an automatic cognitive information processing style, nevertheless they contribute to the perception of the narcissistic person as deceitful, manipulative, and cunning. Horowitz (1975) described a specific type of information processing that involves the use of "sliding meanings." The narcissistic individual tends to disguise or distort information and observations of reality to protect the inflated self-image (see chapter 4 this volume).

For the purpose of this historical account, I here briefly discuss the two most influential theoretical conceptualizations within psychoanalysis, those of Kernberg and Kohut, because their groundbreaking contributions have served to organize and widen the discussion of narcissistic disorders. I also discuss a more recent and less well-known interpersonal approach outlined by Fiscalini (1994; Fiscalini & Grey, 1993), which moved away from the common diagnostic spectrum and identified narcissism based on an interactive model of coparticipant inquiry. Finally, I discuss the role of shame in the formation of personality psychopathology, which were specifically relevant for further understanding of narcissistic functioning and its descriptive features.

The Ego-Psychological and Object Relation Approach   O. Kernberg's (1975, 1980, 1998a) conception of NPD is based on ego psychology and object relations. Inspired by the Kleinian school and specifically by Rosenfeld, Kernberg differentiated pathological narcissism both from normal adult narcissism and from a regression to infantile narcissism in adult individuals. According to his theory, the central etiological factor is the presence of unintegrated early rage, which causes the splitting and projection of the devalued self and object representations from the idealized ones. Together, the idealized self and object representations form the pathological grandiose self lead to the development of a dysfunctional superego that tends to be overly aggressive and often dissociated and projected. Kernberg outlined three areas in which narcissistic character traits can manifest: (1) pathological self-love expressed in grandiosity, superiority, emotional shallowness, and a discrepancy between exaggerated talents and ambitions and actual capacity and achievements; (2) pathological object love characterized by envy and devaluation of others, exploitative behavior, lack of empathy, and inability to depend on others; and (3) superego pathology that can be expressed as an inability to experience depression, severe mood swings, shame-regulated self-esteem, and superficial or self-serving values. More severe superego pathology leads to the syndrome of malignant narcissism, characterized by antisocial behavior, paranoid ideation, and ego-syntonic aggression and sadism. O. Kernberg's (1998b) conceptualization has greatly influenced the definition of NPD in the *DSM* system and has also contributed to generic and unique understanding of narcissistic aspects of organizational development and leadership.

So far, Kernberg's has been the most useful perspective applicable to a broad variety of phenomena ranging from healthy love relationships to severe personality pathology, severe sadistic and criminal behavior, and dysfunctional group and organizational processes.

The Self Psychological Approach   Kohut (1971, 1972, 1977), founder of the self psychological school, identified narcissistic pathology as an arrest in normal narcissistic and self-object development. According to Kohut, narcissism represents a separate developmental line originating from an archaic grandiose self and moving toward the internalization of an ego-ideal and into increased self-cohesion and more mature transformations of narcissism, including healthy self-esteem. Empathic failures lead to arrests in the normal transformation of narcissism. Based on extensive psychoanalytic work with narcissistic patients, Kohut identified two themes that represent needs, fantasies, and expectations derived from an arrested developmental stage dominated by an archaic grandiose self. In therapy these themes are represented by two major types of transference: (1) a mirror transference representing a need for affirmation and approval and (2) an idealizing transference in which the therapist is idealized. In the arrested state, the narcissistic individual is left searching for such mirroring and idealized self-objects. Instead of offering descriptive diagnostic criteria for NPD, Kohut suggested these specific transference developments as diagnostic indicators of narcissistic disorders. He defined primary and secondary types of self-disorders based upon the level of self-cohesion. Among the primary self-disorders, Kohut identified as analyzable the narcissistic behavior disorder, which features temporary breakups or distortions of the self, with reversible symptoms, and NPD, also with temporary self-distortions but with symptoms that involve the person's entire psychological state. Kohut's focus on understanding the specific logic of the patient's inner experiences and his emphasis on empathy as both an observational instrument and a curative tool have made his work very influential in the development of psychoanalytic and psychodynamic techniques in the treatment of narcissistic patients.

The Interpersonal Approach   The interpersonal approach has been represented by Fiscalini (1994; Fiscalini & Grey, 1993), who suggested that narcissism is "a central dimension of psychopathology that cuts across the diagnostic spectrum" (Fiscalini, 1994, p. 749), ranging from milder to more severe forms. He identified two types of narcissism: a defensive characterological type similar to self-centeredness that represents an abnormal development caused by experiences of interpersonal shaming and spoiling, and an archaic developmental narcissism that is more natural and represents early interpersonal needs. According to the interpersonalists, narcissism is a way of protecting a fragile and narcissistically injured interpersonal self. They apply an active method of coparticipant inquiry to explore both the evolving narcissistic transference–countertransference matrix as well as the real nonnarcissistic therapeutic relationship. The idea of "living through a real relationship" refers to the experience of a new and curative formation of a nonnarcissistic relationship. Very few have discussed narcissism with Fiscalini's technical sensitivity and awareness of nuances in clinical expressions, dynamic meanings, and developmental contexts. His work is uniquely helpful in understanding the many potential pitfalls in treatment of narcissistic patients when the therapist/analyst may use poorly timed, excessively confrontational, or overly empathic interventions that fail to address core narcissistic issues for the patient. Learning to meaningfully balance empathy, confrontation, exploration, and interpretations while actively using one's own countertransference is the interpersonalist's avenue toward change in narcissistic experiences and relativeness.

Studies on Shame and Affect Regulation   The role of shame in pathological narcissism and the development of the self have been discussed more intensively among psychoanalysts. Broucek (1982) believed that shame is the most prominent affect in narcissistic personalities and that the grandiose self is posited as a compensatory formation generated in large part by primitive shame experiences. Morrison (1983) also highlighted the central role of shame in narcissistic pathology, both being closely entangled with each other and shame causing narcissistic vulnerability and retreat. Intense shame leads to disruption of narcissistic functioning that can be experienced as hurtful, with feelings of anger and a lowering of self-esteem (Morrison, 1989). Social psychological studies of self-conscious emotions have helped clarify the nature and specific functions of shame in particular but also of envy and empathy, both of which are central to both healthy and pathological narcissism (Tangney & Fischer, 1995). Of importance for the role of shame in pathological narcissism are its associations to low and variable self-esteem, splitting, and impaired capacity for other-oriented empathy and tendencies to hide. The suggestion of a second type of NPD, the shy type (Akhtar, 1997; Cooper, 1998;

Gabbard, 1989), in addition to the arrogant, exhibitionistic type, reflects the significance of the role of shame in addition to aggression in narcissistic pathology. In addition, integrational studies of affect regulation and self-development (Fonagy, Gergely, Jurist, & Target, 2002; Schore, 1994) have added to the understanding of patterns in early life that are central to development of normal and pathological narcissism (see chapter 3 this volume). Findings in early development of shame as an affect regulator, the capacity for mentalization as a precursor for empathic processing, and attachment patterns that affect self-esteem regulation have been central for understanding narcissism.

The Biosocial Learning Perspective

As part of a comprehensive and systematic theory of personality and psychopathology based on a biosocial learning perspective, Millon (1981, 1996, 1998) outlined a matrix of narcissistic personality characteristics capturing several clinical domains, including both overt (expressive, cognitive, and interpersonal) and hidden (self-image and defensive functions) areas of functioning. He also elaborated a set of narcissistic personality subtypes (see above) ordered in sequence of severity. Influenced by Freud's description of the narcissistic libidinal type and by W. Reich's conceptualization of the phallic-narcissistic disorder, Millon specifically highlighted the inflated sense of self-worth and self-admiration in narcissistic individuals; their confident, haughty, and exploitative interpersonal style; their expansive cognitive functioning; and their tendency to rationalize and return to a compensatory and comforting fantasy world when faced with failures or obstacles. Millon's personality theory and characteristics, organized for empirical purposes in the diagnostic self-report MCMI (Millon et al., 1996), has stimulated an enormous amount of research on personality disorders around the world.

The Cognitive Perspective

From a cognitive perspective, Beck, Freeman, and associates (1990) proposed that NPD should be conceived in terms of dysfunctional schemas about the self, the world, and the future. Such schemas reflect beliefs that develop during childhood and persist throughout life, influencing views, reactions, and behaviors in relation both to others and oneself. Young (1994) suggested three core operating schema moods in narcissistic individuals: entitlement, emotional deprivation, and defectiveness. Additional secondary schemas include approval seeking, unrelenting standards, subjugation, mistrust, and avoidance. These maladaptive schemas are further grouped into three clusters that represent separate aspects of the self. In the "special self" mood, the narcissist is superior, entitled, critical, and unempathic. The "vulnerable child" mood is triggered by aloneness, criticism, and failure; the special self is lost, and the narcissist feels empty, humiliated, and ignored and can even become demoralized, self-critical, and depressed. The "self-soother" mood provides a means of avoiding the negative affect of the vulnerable self and serves to detach or numb the narcissist through drugs, excessive work, sex, gambling, or fantasies. The narcissistic patient is assumed to alternate among these three modes when reacting to changes and events in the environment (Young, 1998).

An Empirical Social Psychological Perspective

The most recent contribution to the conceptualizations of narcissistic functioning is based on extensive psychological research over the past two decades on narcissism, self-esteem, and self-regulation using the Narcissistic Personality Inventory (Raskin & Hall, 1979, 1981; Raskin & Terry, 1988; see below). Initially, a series of studies validated the construct of narcissism as associated with a broad range of traits, such as sensation seeking (disinhibition), experience seeking, and boredom susceptibility (Emmons, 1981); uniqueness and extraversion (Emmons, 1984); egocentricity and affect intensity and variability (Emmons, 1987); use of first-person singular pronouns (Raskin & Shaw, 1988); assertiveness and hypercompetitiveness (Watson, Morris, & Miller, 1998); and expressed anger (McCann & Biaggio, 1989). One study also confirmed the negative correlation between narcissism and empathy (Watson, Grisham, Trotter, & Biderman, 1984). In an effort to connect these empirical measures with clinical accounts on narcissism, Raskin and Terry (1988) concluded that "narcissism represents a syndrome of relatively diverse behavior" (p. 899). They identified seven components of narcissism: authority, self-sufficiency, exhibitionism, superiority, vanity, exploitativeness, and entitlement. Accordingly, people who have high narcissism tend to be dominant, extraverted, exhibitionistic, aggressive, impulsive, self-centered, subjectively self-satisfied, self-indulgent, and nonconforming. Raskin, Novacek, and Hogan (1991) went a step further by introducing the first model of narcissistic self-esteem regulation. They suggested that hostility, grandiosity, dominance, and narcissism are all interrelated but also related to variations in self-esteem. In other words, people with high narcissism defend their heightened self-esteem by managing hostility via their grandiose self-representation and interpersonal dominance.

Other researchers exploring self-esteem have joined this avenue of studies on narcissism. One group connected self-esteem regulation to narcissism, ego threats, and aggression (Baumeister, Heatheron, & Tice, 1993; Baumeister, Smart, & Boden, 1996; Bushman & Baumeister, 1998), and another investigated stability and fluctuations in self-esteem and the role of narcissism in the evaluation of and reactions to interpersonal feedback (Kernis, Cornell, Sun, Berry, & Harlow, 1993; Kernis, Grannemann, & Barclay, 1989; Kernis & Sun, 1994). An additional important conjunction was from the studies on self-perception and self-evaluation that looked at the role of narcissism on self-enhancement (John & Robins, 1994; Robins & John, 1997).

Rhodewalt and Morf (1995, 1998; Morf & Rhodewalt, 1993) added to this research a specific interest in cognitive affective aspects of reactions and mood variability in response to failures and success. This led to the proposal of a thorough, empirically substantiated model for narcissism identified as a dynamic self-regulatory process (Morf & Rhodewalt, 2001; Rhodewalt & Sorrow, 2003). They suggested that the narcissistic individual's self develops in a dynamic interactive context of cognitive, motivational, affective, and self-evaluating *intrapersonal* processes that underlie or motivate *interpersonal* behavior and specific self-regulatory strategies vis-à-vis other people. Narcissistic functioning involves strivings for continuous self-affirmation to maintain and enhance the self. The "narcissistic self-concept" is grandiose, that is, inflated and overly positive. Narcissistic individuals use self-enhancing or aggrandizing strategies to maintain high self-esteem and fend off threats toward the self from others. They use self-serving evaluating strategies to exaggerate their own accomplishments and contributions. The self-concept is also unstable because of the narcissistic individuals' emotional hyperresponsiveness, unstable sense of self-worth, and variability in self-esteem, which is highly dependent on how they are perceived in the moment. Narcissistic self-regulation involves perpetuating efforts to elicit and manipulate interpersonal relations and distort feedback. Strategies include interpersonal interactions that serve to maintain a desired identity by avoiding or annulling negative feedback and by soliciting positive feedback from others to preserve external self-affirmation. Interpersonal relationship strategies serve to reinforce the self-concept as the narcissistic individuals not only tend to choose relationships and social context that support and enhance their selves but also intentionally influence the interpersonal or social situation in the service of self-promotion or enhancement of self-esteem. Soliciting admiration and constraining or manipulating others' views to obtain a desired self-image are examples of such strategies. In other words, people with high narcissism are strongly motivated to make positive self-distortions and exaggerate self-attributions in relationships with others.

In addition, narcissistic individuals use various strategies to protect the self at the expense of others. They tend to devalue, derogate, or blame others, and they respond to threatening feedback with anger and hostility. Other examples of interactive strategies are biased interpretations of feedback, selective attention, and selective or distorted recall of past events. A specific strategy, self-handicapping behavior, serves to protect public image as the individual identifies impediments to performance, which are used either to discount subsequent failure or to reinforce success.

Rhodewalt and colleagues concluded that narcissistic functioning leads to interpersonal problems and to a negative cycle that ends in rejection and hostility. Negative views of others, insensitivity to social constraints, hypervigilance, competitiveness, enhancing self-crediting for successes, and aggressive reactions and blaming when failing are all aspects of narcissistic self-regulation that make interpersonal relationships particularly strenuous and threatening. The dynamics of these self-regulatory processes have been related to clinical diagnostic traits for narcissism such as self-exaggeration, arrogant behavior, hostility, entitlement, and lack of empathy. This avenue of very interesting and important research has become increasingly clinically relevant and has opened the door for the much-needed empirical exploration and validation of specific narcissistic dynamics and features.

Research on Narcissistic Personality Disorder

Our knowledge of narcissism and narcissistic disorders stems mostly from three major areas of inquiry: (1) individual case studies of treatment of narcissistic people in psychoanalysis and dynamic psychotherapy, (2) empirical studies of personality disorders in the domain of psychopathology using structured and semistructured diagnostic instruments for evaluating the presence of characteristics of narcissistic patients in psychiatric settings, and (3) studies in the field of academic social psychology (mentioned above) using laboratory experiments and inventories for exploring specific narcissistic traits and behavior.

The introduction of NPD in *DSM-III* in 1980 was to a large extent based on the extensive psychoanalytic studies and formulations, especially Kernberg's and Kohut's contributions. The adaptation of a discrete set of diagnostic criteria led to its inclusion in official diagnostic instruments and in empirical studies of the Axis II personality disorders. Most structured interviews, self-questionnaires, and inventories for personality disorders also include evaluation of narcissistic criteria. This has gradually inspired empirical studies of NPD, which specifically helped to establish differential diagnoses and distinguish NPD from other mental disorders. Despite this, it has been challenging to create an empirical base for defining NPD (Gunderson, Ronningstam, & Smith, 1991). The complex nature of this disorder—high level of functioning, lack of symptoms or consistent behavioral signifiers, hidden or denied intrapsychic problems (even when severe), and lack of motivation to seek psychiatric treatment out of shame, pride, or self-aggrandizing denial—have made it difficult to identify people in general psychiatric settings who meet the *DSM* criteria for NPD. Consequently, funding for psychiatric research on NPD has been less publicly urgent, especially compared with the antisocial personality disorders (ASPD) and BPD, for which more obvious human suffering and extensive social and mental health costs have impelled research on their etiology, course, and treatment.

The Austen Riggs and McLean Hospital Studies

Despite difficulties in NPD research, two series of studies of clinically well-defined narcissistic patients have been conducted, at the Austen Riggs Center and McLean Hospital. The first, by Erik Plakun in the 1980s (Plakun, 1987, 1989, 1990), used data from a long-term follow-up study including medical records and self-administered questionnaires from people who had been in long-term treatment at the Center. In this study, Plakun confirmed the validity of NPD diagnosis vis-à-vis BPD, schizophrenia, and major affective disorder. He also identified a group of patients with unusually severe NPD, with histories of long inpatient treatment and several rehospitalizations. Compared to BPD, this group of severe narcissistic patients had lower social and global functioning at follow-up, more rehospitalizations, and lower levels of subjective satisfaction and less capacity for recovery in midlife. He also found that self-destructive behavior in NPD was associated with poor social functioning at follow-up.

In the other series of studies, at McLean Hospital, the author in collaboration with John Gunderson and colleagues developed the first semi-structured diagnostic interview, the Diagnostic Interview for Narcissism (DIN; Gunderson, Ronningstam, & Bodkin, 1990; see the appendix to this volume), specifically designed for studying pathological narcissism in psychiatric patients. People in inpatient or outpatient treatment with clinically well-established diagnoses of pathological narcissism and NPD were interviewed and compared to others with a broad range of related psychiatric disorders (BPD, ASPD, bipolar disorder, anorexia, and all other psychiatric patients; Gunderson & Ronningstam, 2001; Ronningstam, 1992; Ronningstam & Gunderson, 1989, 1990a, 1991; Stormberg, Ronningstam, Gunderson, & Tohen, 1998). These studies contributed to a delineation of pathological narcissism and helped identify diagnostic criteria for NPD that proved useful for the development of the *DSM-IV* criteria set for NPD (Gunderson, Ronningstam, & Smith, 1991, 1996). The DIN has later been adapted both for adolescents (Adolescent Adaptation to Record Review of [DIN]; P. Kernberg, Hajal, & Normandin, 1998) and for preadolescents (P-DIN; Guile et al., 2004). In a first prospective follow-up study, we found that narcissistic patients changed over time and that corrective life events, that is, achievements, new durable relationships, and disillusionments, contributed to such changes (Ronningstam, Gunderson, & Lyons, 1995). Notable is that in both these series of studies at McLean and Austen Riggs, the participating narcissistic patients had clinically well-identified diagnoses of NPD and pathological narcissism from multiple diagnostic sources over an extended workup period.

Studies on *DSM-IV* NPD Criteria

Revisions of the *DSM* Axis II have over the years significantly improved the criteria set for NPD, and although some of the criteria still fail in specificity, for example, grandiose fantasies and entitlement, the NPD criteria seem to adequately capture the central features of pathological narcissism. Empirical studies provide support for the content validity and discriminating capacity of these criteria. Blais, Hilsenroth, and Castlebury (1997) found in their factor analytic study that grandiosity is a core feature for NPD and that three domains underlie pathological narcissism: grandiosity in fantasy and behavior, need for admiration, and lack of empathy. When compared to the near neighbors ASPD and BPD, the unique criteria for NPD were grandiosity, belief in being special and unique, needing admiration, entitlement, and arrogant and haughty behavior (Holdwick, Hilsenroth, Castlebury, & Blais, 1998). The *DSM-IV* criteria distinguish NPD from BPD, whereas both studies indicate a relationship between NPD and ASPD or sociopathy. Interpersonally exploitative behavior, lack of empathy, and envy were shared with ASPD in Holdwick and colleague's study, and Blais and colleagues identified a sociopathic component consisting of lack of empathy, exploitation, envy, and grandiosity. The author (Ronningstam & Gunderson, 1989) found high discriminating ability for five *DSM-III-R/DSM-IV* criteria: exaggeration of talents, uniqueness, grandiose fantasies, entitlement, and need for admiration. Morey and Jones (1998), on the other hand, were more critical and concerned about the low internal consistency, empirical incoherence, and high diagnostic overlap in the *DSM* criteria. They argued for radical changes, adding reactions to threats to self-esteem, need for interpersonal control, interpersonal hostility, and lack of self-destructive tendencies to the future list of criteria.

The general limitations of *DSM-IV* Axis II in capturing the full range of personality pathology and failing to identify patients whom clinicians consider having personality disorder diagnoses have been pointed out by Westen and Arkowitz-Westen (1998) and by Gunderson, Ronningstam, and Smith (1991). This is particularly consequential for NPD. People with traits of pathological narcissism that range beyond the *DSM-IV* criteria set, or people who have less severe and overt narcissistic pathology and for various reasons do not meet the *DSM-IV* criteria for NPD, will not be correctly identified. In addition, the conceptual meaning and dynamic expressions of several of the concepts, such as entitlement, empathy, and exploitativeness, are unclear and poorly defined, and the interaction between interpersonal interactions, self-esteem fluctuations, and affect dysregulation remains unclear.

The specific nature of pathological narcissism with grandiosity and sensitivity to threats to self-esteem makes self-assessment and one-time diagnostic evaluations with direct inquiries in structured interviews less reliable (Rhodewalt & Morf, 1995; Hilsenroth, Handler, & Blais, 1996). Questions on narcissistic themes may evoke defensive reactions (Gunderson, Ronningstam, & Bodkin, 1990) because narcissistic people make more or less conscious efforts to present themselves in an optimal and favorable way in the service of self-esteem regulation. The nature of some specific narcissistic characteristics, such as self-conscious emotions of shame and envy, which are often hidden or bypassed (Tangney, 1995) and therefore inaccessible to immediate diagnostic evaluation, adds further difficulties in empirical evaluations. In addition, the origin and range of impairments in empathic processing as a personality disorder characteristic, one of the core narcissistic interpersonal features, have so far been insufficiently empirically explored to warrant accurate diagnostic assessment.

Similar problems with assessment using structured methods and self-reports have been observed in the research on people with psychopathy (Hart & Hare, 1998) because of their unreliability as self-informants. Hart noticed that self-report measures of psychopathy proved to be more useful and reliable in studies of "normal" nonpatient populations. This has also been the case for social psychological studies of narcissism in nonclinical samples using the Narcissistic Personality Inventory (Raskin & Terry, 1988) and observations of narcissistic functioning of normal adults in laboratory settings.

Other Studies on Narcissism

Parallel efforts to study narcissism were using self-reports—the MCMI (Millon et al., 1996) and the Narcissistic Personality Inventory (Raskin & Hall, 1979, 1981; Raskin & Terry, 1988)—to examine narcissistic personality styles and behavior. Both of these methods proved sensitive to identify certain aspects of narcissistic character function and have generated substantial and valuable research results. The MCMI was adjusted to the changes in *DSM-III-R* and *DSM-IV* and evaluates the egotistical, self-confident, superior, disdainful, and exploitative behavior of narcissistic people. It has been translated into more than 15 languages and is used widely in clinical personality disorder studies.

The Narcissistic Personality Inventory is a 40-item self-questionnaire that is intended to measure narcissism in nonclinical populations. Narcissism is identified in terms of leadership/authority, superiority/arrogance, self-absorption/self-admiration, and vulnerability/sensitivity (Emmons, 1984), and both healthy and maladaptive aspects of narcissism are captured (Rhodewalt & Morf, 1995). Despite the fact that research studies using the Narcissistic Personality Inventory were conducted mostly on nonclinical samples, the results, especially regarding self-esteem and affect regulation, have proved increasingly relevant and applicable to the understanding of exaggerated and pathological narcissistic functioning. These efforts have been integrated into a dynamic self-regulatory processing model for narcissism functioning by Morf and Rhodewalt (2001; see above).

Research using the Rorschach method to assess NPD proved that certain variables such as reflection and idealization, aggression scores, egocentricity index, and grandiosity could differentiate NPD patients from other personality disorders, especially from the near neighbor BPD and ASPD (Gacono, Meloy, & Berg, 1992; Gacono, Meloy, & Heaven, 1990; Hilsenroth, Fowler, Padawer, & Handler, 1997; Hilsenroth, Hibbard, Nash, & Handler, 1993).

Publications

Several important publications updating clinical and empirical progress have appeared. A special issue of *Psychiatric Clinics of North America* (O. Kernberg, 1989b) was the first major effort to integrate clinical, psychoanalytic, and psychiatric research contributions to the field. In 1990, Erik Plakun published an anthology that also covered both psychoanalytic conceptualization and case discussion, and empirical research on narcissistic patients. Several psychoanalytic volumes specifically address identification and treatment of narcissistic patients (Grundberger, 1971; Rothstein, 1980; Bach, 1985; Morrison, 1989; Sandler, Person, & Fonagy, 1991; Masterson, 1993; Fiscalini & Grey, 1993; Giovaccini, 2000). The author's edited volume *Disorders of Narcissism—Diagnostic, Clinical, and Empirical Implications* (Ronningstam, 1998), now translated into both Japanese and Italian, includes discussions of different theoretical perspectives and new treatment modalities, as well as an overview of the accumulating empirical research. Several practical handbooks on dealing with narcissistic individuals and problems in the corporate workplace by Maccoby (2002) and N. W. Brown (2002), and in couples and families by Solomon (1989), Donaldson-Pressman and Pressman (1994), and N. W. Brown (2001), have added to a broader understanding of narcissistic behavior and interpersonal relativeness. In addition, a practical semi-autobiographical handbook with accompanying informative web sites was written by a layperson, Sam Vaknin (1999)

Conclusions

This historical overview of narcissism describes an unusual development of inquiry and observations, beginning in literature and art, developing within psychoanalytic thinking, and presently being reconsidered in empirical psychological and psychosocial research. Few psychiatric or psychoanalytic concepts lend themselves to such broad array of connotations and associations. This overview outlines a gradual integration of ideas and techniques of inquiry from different fields, which it is hoped will promote increased clarification and understanding of narcissism. It also points to future research and areas of new clinical advances.

2

A Normal Asset With Cultural Differences

Normal Narcissism

The extensive interest in disordered narcissism has usually overshadowed studies of narcissistic functioning within what can be considered the normal range. Less is known about the overall vicissitudes within and interactions between normal healthy and exceptional forms of narcissism and how they contrast or interweave in an individual with depreciated or pathological narcissism. Likewise, the importance of normal narcissistic functioning for individual mental health and capacity to live an optimal life has mostly been taken for granted. Healthy narcissistic functions, such as a sense of the right to one's own life, striving for the best in life, appreciation of health and beauty, and ability to compete as well as to protect and defend oneself, are usually first attended to when they are absent or noticed as extreme. Nevertheless, healthy narcissism plays a crucial role in the human capacity to manage challenges, successes, and changes; to overcome defeats, illnesses, trauma, and losses; to love and be productive and creative; and to experience happiness, satisfaction, and acceptance of the course of one's life.

In a broad sense, narcissism refers to feelings and attitudes toward one's own self and to normal development and self-regulation. It is the core of normal healthy self-esteem, affects, and relationships. In psychoanalytic terms, normal narcissism is defined as a positive investment in a normally functioning self-structure. Freud's (1914/1957) original thoughts on narcissism are still most relevant for our present understanding of normal narcissistic functioning and how it may differ from the pathological versions. He suggested that narcissism represents a normal developmental line that leads to obtaining new intrapsychic structures. The "ego-ideal" (p. 94) is the central constituent of normal narcissism and the aim of a person's normal self-love. The ego-ideal represents what one wants to be or accomplish in life and what one compares and measures one's actual self against. It is based on identification with parents or others who have been idealized. Another aspect of normal narcissism is self-regard. In "self-regard" Freud included the experience of being loved by others as well as having one's love returned and possessing the loved object. While such experiences increase self-regard and self-esteem, being in love, on the contrary, and loving someone else challenges or lowers self-regard. "A person in love is humble. A person who loves has, so to speak, forfeited a part of his narcissism, and it can only be replaced by his being loved" (p. 98). However, the inability to love is a source of inferiority feelings. Freud also included in self-regard the success in achieving whatever ambitions and goals the ego-ideal sets that help increase the self-regard. For Freud, the third aspect of normal narcissism was related to the development of object relations, and involved "narcissistic object choice" (p. 98), that is, the choice of another with the aim of being loved by that person.

Self-preservation and Normal Entitlement

The function of healthy self-regard has been associated with self-preservation and normal entitlement. Stone (1998) describes "self-preservation" as the instinct to survive, to protect and defend oneself, to look out for the best for oneself, to evaluate oneself and adjust one's goals based on a realistic self-evaluation, to do the best and make the most of one's life in the areas of both love and work. The capacity to form and maintain gratifying relationships—friendships as well as intimate relationships—is another aspect of self-preservation linked to preservation of the human being, to guarantee the survival of present and coming generations.

While entitlement usually refers to social, political, and economic rights and opportunities, a broad range of normal narcissistic rights and expectations are associated with emotional entitlement. Such entitlement involves the right to feeling satisfied, special, and unique; to be and do the best; to accomplish, win, and be celebrated; to be acknowledged and the center of attention; and to have the right to expect attention, respect, and support when asked for and needed. A sense of entitlement can also be an important motivational force in an individual's personal and professional development.

Due to its association to pathological narcissism, that is, to unrealistic expectations and exaggerated overbearing interpersonal demandingness, entitlement as a fundamentally healthy aspect of normal narcissism and normal life functioning tends to be easily disregarded. Regular conflicts of entitlement involve perceptual differences regarding rights, duties, privileges and obligations, and a perception of the disrespectful and tactless use of someone's time and space (Pierce, 1978). These conflicts are usually accompanied by self-righteousness and feelings of anger and envy. When representing a psychological phenomenon, normal entitlement refers to an inner experience of oneself as an agent of one's own intentions and actions, and to expectations of predictable and reasonable responses. In other words, entitlement is related to a sense of having the right to one's interpersonal and intrapersonal space and to one's own feelings and thoughts, and it is rooted in a deep feeling of deserving what is meant, done, and possible for oneself. Conflicts of such entitlement, which may require extensive exploration to discern, are usually associated to feelings of shame or rage. A sense of psychological entitlement develops during childhood foremost in the early interaction between parents and child (Kriegman, 1983; Moses & Moses-Hrushovski, 1990; Stone 1998).

Case vignette

Amanda, 7 years old, reminded her father at breakfast that he forgot to say good night to her last night and told him that she felt neglected and hurt. The father apologized, explaining that he had been doing the taxes, gave her an extra morning hug, and promised that he would not forget her again. Another child, 7-year-old Clara, whose mother also forgot to say good night last night because she had too many drinks in the afternoon and was drunk at the time of her daughter's bedtime, did not remind her mother next morning. She assumed that the mother was not feeling well and had learned from past experiences of her mother's irritable reactions not to intrude when the mother needed to be alone.

While Amanda obviously expected that her feelings and reactions would be acknowledged by her father, Clara's sense of emotional entitlement was much more compromised.

Kriegman (1983) differentiated among normal entitlement, exaggerated entitlement, and restricted or "nonentitlement" and suggested that human beings manifest all three types. Exaggerated entitlement, usually associated with pathological narcissism, involves more or less overtly expressed inordinate or unrealistic ideas and feelings of deserving excessive rights and expectations. Nonentitlement, less acknowledged as a narcissistic disturbance and more difficult to discern, refers to an ego-syntonic inability to identify and express certain rights, desires, and expectations, resulting in overt self-righteous indignation and underlying feelings of worthlessness. People with restricted or compromised entitlement may form idealized relationships with idealized other(s) with the expectation that if they do the right thing and reach the other's approval or love they may be given what they expect. Usually they end up disappointed.

Entitlement serves an important part in normal self-esteem regulation. However, in pathological narcissism with self-esteem dysregulation, entitlement is exaggerated and associated with boastful grandiosity, and it serves to modulate underlying feelings of inferiority, shame, and rage. Exaggerated and restricted entitlement can often coexist, the former being a compensation for the latter. For example, when people feel not entitled or unable to express what they want but expect others to figure out their wishes, they get upset if their expectations are not properly met. Restricted entitlement can be confused with modesty, which is a culturally determined aspect of narcissistic functioning (Stone, 1998). Modesty represents the balance between feelings of deserving and the socially acceptable norms for self-referential and entitled behavior.

Self-reference

Expressions of pride and self-fulfillment can range from strikingly exhibitionistic attention- seeking behavior, to modest, reserved attitudes, even including tendencies to shun attention. Not only personal differences, but also contextual circumstances and cultural values and customs play major roles in such self-manifestations. Compare the exuberant joy and exultant satisfaction of an extraverted intense young leader of a rock band who finally reaches his dream of performing at a concert for 25,000 people, with the reserved satisfaction of a shy, introverted collector of rare stamps who after years of searching is able to add an exceptional stamp to his collection. Or the following "peak reactions" to a successful ascent of a mountain: while the British climber calmly stated, "The mountain graciously opened its doors to us and we had the privilege of ascending its peak," two American climbers were simultaneously jumping around, hugging each other, and ecstatically screaming, "We made it!!!!"

The sports arena, one of the most competitive and success-focused activities in our society, reveals great personal variations in self-referential behavior. Bonnie Blair, the former speed-skating champion, was praised for her unique combination of confidence and competitiveness, unassuming manner, modesty and camaraderie, and especially her capacity to show concern and encouragement to those defeated. At the opposite end of the scale is Mohammed Ali, the former heavyweight boxing world champion, whose outlandish, boisterous self-promoting and self-aggrandizing behavior was featured worldwide. Nevertheless, after ending his boxing career and developing Parkinson's disease, Ali underwent a remarkable modification of his extreme self-centeredness. Utilizing his world recognition, he began promoting world peace and received the 1997 Peace and Tolerance Prize from the Jewish-Arab Center for Peace. These examples indicate not only the range of individual presentations from unpretentiousness and humility to extreme self emphasizing and promoting behavior, but also the changeability in such personal narcissistic characteristics that can be influenced and modified by life events and corrective personal life experiences (see chapter 8 this volume).

Empathy

Empathy is often taken for granted. Like electricity, its presence is invisible, and it is usually noticed first by its absence. Empathy is an essential aspect of narcissistic functioning and self-esteem regulation, because it involves several internal abilities for evaluating and understanding other peoples' inner experiences and feelings. Because empathy represents the capacity to feel what another person feels, it is crucial to an individual's sense of mastering interpersonal relationships and social interactions. Empathy refers to the ability to feel and perceive the inner psychological state of others, and it requires a role-taking capacity and the ability to identify the feelings and needs of other people. In addition, it requires the ability to feel one's own emotions (Feshbach, 1975). Also included is the capacity to form hypotheses about and identify with others' feelings and experiences, and to separate oneself from one's own feelings in order to not only react to the other's feelings, but to be able to evaluate the origin and significance of the other's emotions within the experienced context (Basch, 1983; Tangney, 1991, 1995). Empathy is paradoxically related to the capacity for self-comforting and tolerating one's own distress and negative feelings, especially shame. The ability to modulate negative affects and to shift into a positive state enables the process of empathy (Schore, 1994). The capacity for empathy is compromised by shame feelings because of their accompanying urge to withdraw and hide (Tangney, 1995).

Empathy evolves with the neuropsychological development and the child's acquiring of cognitive and ego capacities. The capacity for empathy has its neurological base located in the frontal lobe with the dorsolateral frontal systems involving the cognitive aspects of empathic processing and the orbitofrontal systems involving the emotional empathic processing (Eslinger, 1998). Based on studies of deficits in empathic capacity in learning-disabled children, Garber (1989) identified certain cognitive integrative skills that are essential for immediate and accurate empathic responses. He stated that "empathy involves reasoning with the other's unconscious affect and experiencing his experiences with him while the empathizer maintains the integrity of his self intact" (p. 621). Resources necessary for object-centered empathy include "memory, fantasy, conceptualization and other cognition in relation to impulses, affects, body sensations, superego pressures and gratifications, defenses, and need-satisfying as well as gratifying introjects. . . . Consequently, the capacity for empathy would require highly developed ego functions such as thought, memory, comprehension, and conceptualization of the purpose of integrating the affective cues" (pp. 621–622).

Fonagy, Gergely, Jurist, and Target (2002) emphasize the interpersonal aspect of empathy as part of the reflective mode called mentalization. They suggest that the capacity to predict and experience the feelings of others, which gradually develops in the early attachment, involves an "interpersonal interpretive mechanism." Because empathy requires the individual to "assume another's perspective and to infer and, to some degree, experience their emotional state of mind" (p. 137), the affect part of this interpretive mechanism is essential and responsible for emotional resonance, that is, empathy.

Empathy differs from sympathy in that sympathy focuses on the similarities between one's own feelings and those of others. Sympathy also involves sharing feelings and feeling along with the other, and persons who sympathize are hence more preoccupied with their own feelings and less tuned in to the understanding of others' feelings.

Self-conscious Emotions

Inasmuch as shame and envy have been considered the weeds in the gar-den of emotions, they are still most pivotal in both healthy and disordered narcissism. While they are fundamentally social and interpersonal, they are also intra-individual. They involve both physiological and behavioral aspects, as well as cognitive appraisals, comparisons, and interpretations of other people and situations. At appropriate levels, these feelings serve important roles promoting more constructive human functioning, as well as socially and personally adaptive behavior (Tangney, 1995). Shame is essential for self-evaluation and self-regulation (Schore, 1994). Feelings of shame can promote awareness and changes in interpersonal relation-ships, foster modesty and concern, improve social standards, and restrain socially detrimental behavior. As such, shame has a signaling function that serves to help the individual both to avoid potentially negative conse-quences and to support psychological well-being (Greenwald & Harder, 1998). Moderate and acceptable envy usually co-occur with feelings of admiration toward the envied person (Habimana & Masse, 2000). Envy can promote self-improvement and help persons to identify what they value, want, and care about, and guide them to communicate such wishes and to access desired possessions, objects, and relationships.

Both feelings—shame and envy—easily go unnoticed because they involve avoidance and self-depreciation. Noticing one's own shame or envy actually triggers both reluctance to admit such feelings and addi-tional feelings of shame because of their association with experiences of inferiority, rejection, and failure (Lansky, 1997). Considered socially undesirable, they are nevertheless socioculturally significant and omni-present in human relationships. In some cultures, envy is considered a sin; in others it is associated with witchcraft and the "evil eye," unex-plainable or malicious aggression or destructiveness, and can even lead to ostracism of or criminal behavior toward the envied person(s). In high shame cultures where people are used to hiding shameful experiences, public exposure may be an extremely humiliating and sometimes deadly punishment.

Shame manifests as a painful feeling of an interrupted sense of joy, rela-tionship, status, or pride, because of exposure of ones failure to meet stan-dards or ideals (Lansky, 1997). It originates in visual interactions and the experience of being looked at by a valued significant other and is reflec-tive of the individual's interpretation of a situation. Shame occurs in the beginning of the second year of life when the toddler is facing unfulfilled expectations and facially expressed affect misattunement (Schore 1998). Shame is "an acutely painful stress-associated affect, [which] triggers a rapid de-energizing state in the infant in which the deflated self, depleted of energy, withdraws, recoils, and attempts to disappear from the view of significant objects" (p. 66). The process of shame is later internalized into the self's negative evaluation of the self, an evaluation that may or may not have been evoked by public exposure (Morrison, 1987; Schore, 1994). In such contexts, feelings of shame can be hidden, bypassed, or unconscious. Shame triggers the urge to withdraw, hide, and not be seen (H. B. Lewis, 1971; Tangney, 1990, 1995). Shame can also serve as a signal and defense, indicating behavior or situations that would lead to feelings of more manifest shame (Lansky, 1997). In addition, shame can evoke anger reactions that may also serve to defend against the painful feelings of shame (Tangney, Wagner, Fletcher, Gramzow, 1992). Embarrassment, the affective component of self-awareness and self-evaluation, is a less intense form of shame (M. Lewis, 1995).

Envy, on the other hand, involves a comparison and admiration of another's superiority, and in normal narcissism, admiration is a gratifying, joyful activity (Sandell, 1993). Envy also involves longing for the desired person or object and the wish to be equal to or surpass that person. The person compares himself or herself, and in this comparison the individual's self-esteem and self-evaluation are threatened either by someone perceived as more successful or better endowed or by the envying person's experience of his or her own value or social position as lowered. What follows is a narcissistic humiliation with feelings of inferiority and decreased self-esteem (Spielman, 1971). Most important, envy is also associated with anger at the desired person and urges to destroy what is seen as good. Manifestations of envy can range from experiences of injustice and unfairness, and feeling cheated, to self-aggrandizing and diminishing of the other's accomplishments, to various maneuvers to devalue and sabotage the desired person's future accomplishments, to narcissistic rage and destructive actions toward that person (Habimana & Masse, 2000; Lansky, 1997). Aggressive envy-related behavior may represent an attempt to protect self-esteem and prevent self-depreciation. In addition, envy can also serve as a defense against unbearable feelings of shame. Feelings of envy are most often disowned and may only be inferred from people's experiences in their interpersonal relationships (Lansky, 1997). Envy may also be projected, as the person believes that others are envious of him or her because of their specialness (Ronningstam & Gunderson, 1990). Jealousy is related to envy but occurs in a triadic situation and involves protective guarding, suspiciousness and rivalry, and fear of loosing affection and love from another to an intruding third person (Spielman, 1971).

Control, Power, and Rage

Because the development of narcissism stems from the experience of infantile omnipotence, normal narcissism is intimately related to a sense of control and mastery. Positive self-esteem and self-regard involve the experience of inner autonomy and sense of control of thoughts, feelings, experiences, and impulses. Stone (1998) considered the psychobiological aspects of aggression and assertive behavior to be similar in both humans and animals, which include survival and protection of one's self and territory, competitive and predatory behavior, and maternal aggressive behavior serving to protect a child. The common denominator for all these behaviors is that they occur within social norms serving to protect continuing life, affiliation, and development of self and others. Kohut (1972) describes the "catastrophic reaction" (p. 383)—a rage reaction related to but not identical with narcissistic rage. This reaction occurs in response to an experience of incapacity, such as the inability to be in control of one's own thought processes, which are some of the most important parts of one's own self. Lack of control, disempowerment, helplessness, and impotence are related to basic entitlement and the rights to safety, reliability, protection, space, and ownership. The rage is triggered by the lack of omnipotence and control and the accompanying feelings of shame. It is important to differentiate this type of rage reaction from violence, destructive competitiveness, sadism, and revengeful aggression.

Grandiose Fantasies or Potential Success

Grandiosity has usually been connected with achievement, recognition, self-exaggeration, superiority, or sense of being special. Talents, beauty, intelligence, personal attributes, wealth, fame, or special positions and family roles are the most common components in the grandiose self-experience and fantasies. In addition, strivings both for perfectionism and for success have been closely associated to narcissism. In adaptive and healthy forms of perfectionism, high standards of performance are linked with feelings of pleasure, sense of competence, experience of freedom, and acceptance of limitations (Blatt, 1995). Perfectionism becomes maladaptive or symptomatic when it serves to compensate for underlying feelings of inferiority and when the major motivation is to avoid failure. Relevant for narcissistic functioning is the distinction between actual strivings for perfectionistic performance in order to seek attention and admiration or acceptance from admired others, versus attempts to create or maintain an inner idealized image of oneself as perfect. The latter represents an omnipotent fantasy and strivings that can be more or less well-anchored in reality. Perfectionism is closely related to the ego-ideal and to vulnerability to criticism. Failure to measure up to standards often results in feelings of shame, especially if the inner standards are set too high (Hollender, 1965; Rothstein, 1980; Hewitt & Flett, 1991).

Success usually increases self-esteem and personal satisfaction. Nevertheless, there is a complex relationship between narcissism and the capacity for reaching and ability to experience success. One of the most important tasks in assessing and understanding narcissism is to differentiate unrealistic and defensive aspects of grandiosity or grandiose fantasies from realistic potentials and competence for successful achievements. However, it is also important to differentiate narcissistic inhibitions and intolerance of success from realistic potentials and competence.

A healthy sense of competence develops in a context of positive self-esteem and talents with predictable feedback and consistent performance criteria. The link between ability and success involves both a capacity to feel and tolerate feelings related to success and the ability to build on positive experiences and accomplishments (Berglas, 1986). For example, fantasizing about winning the Nobel Prize may have a motivating and stimulating function for a hard-working young researcher who just received a major first award for his groundbreaking research results. This is in contrast to the aimless graduate student who never finished his Ph.D. but who is secretly nourishing the idea that some day his unusual talents will be discovered and he will be considered eligible for the Nobel Prize. On the other hand, the Nobel Prize fantasy might contribute to a certain scientific arrogance that could potentially jeopardize a promising research career, whereas for the aimless person such a fantasy could, in the context of a corrective life experience, attach to potential capability and motivation to pursue an area of competence that could be modified into realistic self-evaluation, ambitions, and goals.

The Challenge of Success

Narcissism has usually been discussed in the context of unrealistic ideas of success and the difficulties of tolerating lack of success. Less attention has been paid to the specific experiences and narcissistic challenges involved in facing success, triumphs, and personal victories. The fact that narcissistic functioning may include achievement orientation and attention seeking does not necessarily also imply an ability to sustain the stress and process experiences of real success.

Case vignettes

Ms. G was elected valedictorian of her graduating class. She came from a nonintellectual background and had often heard that she would not amount to much. Starting high school was therefore a specific challenge for Ms. G, and she felt that she had to prove both to herself and to others that she was a capable student with serious ambitions. She was intelligent but also worked hard to get the highest grades. She was considered a "nerd" and a loner but was well respected for her knowledge and ambitions. Ms. G felt extremely anxious and uncomfortable when she realized that as the elected valedictorian she had to deliver the valedictory address at commencement. She felt capable of achieving good grades but shunned the attention of an audience and felt incapable of writing and presenting a speech. She decided to get a ghost writer, and a friend of her cousin who was a college dropout with song-writing ambitions agreed to write the address for her. At the commencement, Ms. G found to her surprise that the address was very well received, and several teachers and students praised her. She was also asked out on dates by a few of the more attractive young men, a new experience. However, after graduation Ms. G began to feel like a fraud. She believed that she did not deserve her nomination and the honor, and she felt guilty for having taken it from someone who could have better matched the ideal image of a valedictorian. She felt lost, and despite the fact that she had been accepted to a good college, she was unable to see college studies as a step forward.

Mr. N, the only son of two lawyers, was a smart and popular high school student for whom knowledge and achievements had come relatively easily. Learning that he had been elected valedictorian of his class, he was very happy and decided to invite all his friends to a party to share his success. In his speech at commencement, he acknowledged the camaraderie and support of his classmates, whom he thought had contributed to a fair and constructive competitive atmosphere in the class. He identified himself as a representative of a group accomplishment and said that he was looking forward to joining some of his classmates in college the next fall. However, it came as a shock for Mr. N when he unexpectedly faced resentment and envy from some of his classmates who refused to share his joy.

Mr. O, an arrogant young man, raised by a single parent for whom his academic achievements meant a lot, graduated magna cum laude from college. On the day of commencement, he felt entitled to park in the dean's parking space. Discovering after commencement that his car had been towed and that he had to pay a fine to get the car back, he had an outburst of rage, stormed into the dean's office, and demanded that his car be delivered back to him immediately.

A success, whether in business, academics, sports, or other professional or personal activities, is a great opportunity for personal change and maturity and for long-term growth. However, it also involves specific challenges, and, paradoxically, such a seemingly desirable event may for many people be experienced as unexpectedly stressful and accompanied by less desirable and even painful feelings. Berglas (1986) describes the "success syndrome," expectations, obligations, and negative stress caused by the ramifications and new conditions following a success. Not only does success require personal changes and accommodations, but also it can lead to interpersonal conflicts and losses, unreasonable and unwanted expectations and requirements, and different disordered behavior related to entitlement, sudden loss of capability, shame, and self-handicapping or sabotaging behavior. Paradoxically, some people can show an escalation of more excessive narcissistic reactions such as extraordinary entitlement and interpersonal hostility. In severe cases, depression, substance abuse, and even suicide may follow.

The question is what makes a success such an opportunity and what may compromise its potential for growth? On a basic structural level, as mentioned above, the presence of normal healthy aggression and approving and guiding superego functioning is essential. On a more specific level, facing a victory involves the capacity for healthy competition and achievement and the presence of healthy entitlement, that is, a genuine feeling that one deserves the distinction and a sense of personal significance. To be able to integrate the experiences of success, a person must be able to tolerate guilt and loneliness while also balancing feelings of separateness, superiority, and pride with feelings of belongingness, gratitude, and concern. In addition, the abilities to enjoy public exposure (exhibitionism), to reciprocate admiring attention, and to tolerate the possibility of envious, critical, or rejecting reactions from others are also crucial.

Cultural Differences in Healthy and Unhealthy Narcissism

East and West

Narcissism and narcissistic disorders have usually been considered phenomena of the Western world. Not only did the studies of narcissism originate in Europe and continue to progress in the United States, but also narcissism has been connected with sociopolitical societies and cultures that emphasize individualism as compared to family, group, or community affiliation. Comparisons between the individualistically, "I-"oriented Western cultures and the collectivistic "we"-oriented Eastern cultures have indicated that Western cultures, which promote inner separateness and independent self-motivation, assertiveness, and mobility, would urge narcissistic functioning and lay the foundation for the development of narcissistic personality disorder (NPD). The international controversy about the existence of NPD and the fact that NPD is not included in WHO's diagnostic system (ICD-10) may have underscored such an impression.

However, the internationally widespread usage of the *DSM* and structured diagnostic interviews has by now to some degree helped to bridge these cultural differences and inspired studies on NPD in other parts of the world, such as Japan, Australia, and Scandinavia. Nevertheless, the culturally biased description of NPD has until recently remained a major obstacle for identifying and studying it in non-Western cultures.

Narcissistic functioning was first defined as overemphasized and exaggerated self-preoccupation, overt grandiosity, exhibitionism, and arrogance, as a self-esteem dysregulation in environments influenced by Western norms and expectations. The introduction of the "hypervigilant," "closet," or "shy" narcissistic personality (Akhtar, 1997; Cooper, 1998;

Gabbard, 1989; Masterson, 1993;) and the new understanding of narcissistic functioning as less overt, more complex, and primarily intrapsychic made the identification of pathological narcissism less dependent on cultural behavior and contexts. In a report on the role of culture in the development of NPD, Warren and Capponi (1995–1996) suggested that the prevalent exhibitionistic form of NPD in the United States has counterparts in the shy narcissist in Japan and Denmark. Moreover, the connection between narcissism and shame (Broucek, 1982; Morrison 1989) contrasting with formulations that relate narcissism mostly to conflicts of unresolved anger, rage, hatred, and envy, has stimulated discussions on narcissism in more shame- dominated cultures, especially Japan.

Japanese Studies

One major difference between Japan and the West with relevance for narcissistic functioning is people's approach to their interpersonal environment. Tatara (1993) formulated this in terms "field dependency," which is the predominant orientation in Japan, and "field independency," which is the preferred interactional mode in the West. The differences are specifically noticeable in interpersonal speech and communication. The Japanese culture emphasizes *how* to speak and say things with specific attention to interpersonal context and subtleties, whereas Western cultures emphasize *what* to say (p. 232). Tatara (1976) also described a tendency among Japanese people to value vagueness and ambiguity in interpersonal relationships and to behave in a way that makes them more ordinary and less noticeable, in other words, more an affiliated member of a group than an outstanding and conspicuous individual.

Studies of pathological narcissism in Japan have been of particular interest because the Western-defined narcissism concept was applied to a specific Japanese psychiatric phenomenon. Several decades of studies on one of the most frequently occurring clinical problems in Japan, *taijin kyofu sho* or anthropophobia, have suggested a link to narcissism as referring to insecure self-esteem. According to Tatara (1993), the major symptoms of *taijin kyofu sho*, that is, intense self-consciousness in close social circles and strong needs to preserve a grandiose self-image and be perceived as unique and visible, stem from a specific interactional pattern between mother and child that is culturally and socioeconomically determined in Japan. The child serves as an extension of the mother, who tends to overprotect and live through her child. As a result, the young person develops a symptom of "'not-to-be-seen' though there is a desperate need 'to-be-seen'" (Tatara, 1993, p. 228). When the child is closely held and protected and expressions of assertiveness and aggression are inhibited, there is a potential for regression in affect and self-image and a risk for violence and suicide. In another growing problem in Japan, the "apathy syndrome" among college students who have lost their capacity to concentrate on their studies, researchers have identified a striking tendency for the students to maintain a grandiose self-image while denying the seriousness of their problems and believing that they actually have the capacity to study if they make an effort and concentrate.

Cultural Tolerance of Shame Versus Anger

The clinical findings on the shy, hypervigilant narcissist show that grandiose desires are usually not expressed and acted upon, and narcissistic pursuits are often performed on a fantasy level. These people suffer from shame, because of their strong wish to exhibit themselves, and guilt, due to the awareness of the inability genuinely and mutually to relate to and care for other people (Cooper & Ronningstam, 1992; Gabbard, 1989). They are usually aware of the discrepancies between their grandiose view of themselves and their capacity and functioning. Such awareness causes intense self-criticism, deep feelings of inferiority and shame, fear of failure in living up to grandiose aspirations, and an inability to appreciate one's own achievements.

A possible relationship between these seemingly irreconcilable views of narcissism, the shame-based narcissism leading to shyness and avoidance, and the aggression-based narcissism leading to assertiveness, exhibitionism, and arrogance, has been suggested in recent research. Studies have shown that feelings of shame can initiate anger, humiliated fury, and hostility. Shame proneness was consistently correlated with anger arousal, suspiciousness, resentment, irritability, a tendency to blame others for negative events, and indirect expression of hostility (Tangney, Wagner, Fletcher, & Gramzow, 1992). The pain of shame and its resulting loss of self-esteem may give rise to unfocused anger and hostility. The aggression is initially directed toward the self. However, shame-based anger can easily be directed toward others as a retaliation, because shame typically involves the imagery of a real or imagined disapproving other (Wicker, Payne, & Morgan, 1983). Unrecognized or unacknowledged shame is likely to result in rage that is directed inward or outward. However, if the person recognizes that the rage is inappropriate or unjust, it may lead to further shame or guilt (H. B. Lewis, 1971).

Cultures differ in their acceptance of and emphasis on both shame and aggression. It is plausible to assume that overt expressions of shame-related aggression can be culturally determined in that certain cultures tolerate or accept expressions of aggression whereas others do not. This may also be true of shyness and individual humility, which in American culture are considered an imposition, like a social handicap. However, in cultures such as those in parts of Scandinavia and Japan, such feelings and attitudes are more readily accepted and even considered a virtue. The overt expressions of narcissistic reactions and pathology will by necessity be influenced by such sociocultural differences. For example, self-assertive or shame-based aggression is more recognized and accepted in the West, leading to a more exhibitionistic, arrogant type of NPD. In the East, on the other hand, the emphasis on holding and covering feelings, including aggression, and modulating assertiveness leads to more internal compromises of narcissistic conflicts and reactions promoting a shy, hypervigilant type. Furthermore, modesty, or a self-restrained and unselfish attitude, is specifically predominant in areas influenced by Buddhism and Lutheranism. Although this may appear totally opposite to narcissism, it is important to identify how living up to such virtues in itself for the individual can be a source of pride and high esteem as well as praise and acknowledgment from others.

Sociocultural Changes

The differences between cultures are also subject to a certain degree of breakup. Cultural changes caused by immigration, technology, and political development can indeed influence both individual narcissistic functioning and the context in which the narcissistic behavior is determined or evaluated. A survey of the European Nordic region (Roberts, 2003), a region that has been identified by anthropologists as relatively introvert and taciturn, reported an ongoing identity change toward increased openness and communicativeness. Finland has by now the highest rates of mobile phones in the world, indicating a boost in human interactions and verbal communication. Similarly, increased awareness in the United States of the consequences of narcissistic leadership and pathological narcissism in the workplace have highlighted a need for corporate cultural changes promoting stronger group affiliation, team collaboration, and loyalty to organizational values and goals. This development will certainly contribute to a continuing productive cross-cultural exploration of normal and pathological narcissism and to an exchange of observations and knowledge between East and West.

Conclusion

This chapter attended to a much neglected area of narcissistic functioning—the normal, healthy and exceptional ways that narcissism in a more or less noticeable way influences our daily life and personal development. Self-conscious emotions such as shame and envy, empathy and entitlement actually constitute important support for normal self-agency and assertiveness. Studies of cultural differences in narcissistic functioning are still relatively speculative and relating to self-esteem regulatory functions in different religious and socio-cultural value systems.

3

The Origins and Scope of Narcissistic Personality Disorder

The Origins of NPD

Until recently, there was a common opinion that parenting pattern contributed to the development of NPD. In the absence of early infant and parent–child interaction studies, and other family studies on the early origin of pathological narcissism and the etiology of adult NPD, each theoretical school derived its own hypothesis about the genesis of pathological narcissism that could explain the later development of NPD. According to the ego psychological object relation theory (O. Kernberg, 1989, 1998), a cold, frustrating parenting style (usually from a mother) with hidden aggression and indifference in an otherwise superficially well-structured environment could implement the development of NPD. The child reacts with aggression, envy, devaluation, and resentment to early parental frustration. These earliest feelings of rage and envy form the core state which the narcissistic individual later defend himself against. Theories pertinent to the self and the "self-system" (Akhtar, 1997; Cooper 1998; Kohut, 1968, 1972) have stressed the lack of match or attunement between parent and child, and the parents' repeated failures to empathically mirror their child's affects and meet the needs of the child leading to a developmental arrest and the development of the grandiose self.

The biosocial learning model for personality disorders (Millon, 1996, 1998; Millon & David, 2000) suggested that being special and overindulgent during childhood leads to the development of NPD. The child acquires a sense of self-sufficiency, values himself or herself regardless of real attainments, and expects to become automatically admired or favored. These experiences lay the foundation for developing a passive self-oriented attitude. Authors representing cognitive theory (Beck, Freeman & Associates, 1990; Young, 1998) also believe in a doting parenting style (i.e., excessively idealizing parenting, usually by the mother) that instills a sense of "specialness" in the child while depriving the child of true affects and fostering a sense of entitlement. The child receives special privileges and treatment but little genuine empathy for his or her real needs and feelings. In addition to a doting mother, there is usually a devaluing, isolated, or detached father, who is devalued and/or critical and rejecting. Often the fathers are successful and overly involved in work (Young, 1998).

Each of these theories has provided valuable ideas about the origin of grandiosity and suggested essential developmental experiences and interactional patterns. Nevertheless, there has been a lack of real understanding of the interaction between normal affect, self-esteem and interpersonal development, and dispositional, experiential, and environmental factors as they relate to and influence narcissism. This chapter describes findings and observations from more recent studies that address the complex nature of narcissistic development and identify the child's age-appropriate and compromised approaches to narcissistic developmental tasks, such as self-regulation, mastering and control, and managing of narcissistic vulnerability.

Heritability

Although NPD has been considered most resistant to change both in psychiatric and psychotherapeutic treatment, the thought of a genetic disposition or vulnerability for development of pathological narcissism has only recently been considered. Two studies have suggested a genetic influence on the development of personality disorders, including NPD. Jang, Livesley, Vernon, and Jackson (1996) found an average of 45% heritability in a study of 483 twin pairs using the Dimensional Assessment of Personality Problems (DAPP-DQ) scale, which captures a basic dimension of narcissism. A more recent study of more than 200 twins (Torgersen et al., 2000) showed that genes could explain nearly 80% of the variation in the trait of NPD. While the meaning and consequences of these findings still await future research, we do know that of specific importance for the development of NPD are inherited variations in hypersensitivity, strong aggressive drive, low anxiety or frustration tolerance, and defects in affect regulation (Schore, 1994).

Neurobiological Origins of Affect Regulation

Parents normally help their children to develop realistic self-esteem and to modulate and neutralize grandiosity, narcissistic distress, and excitement. However, inconsistent attunement and insufficient attachment can lead to failure in the development of functioning self-esteem and affect regulation. Schore (1994) suggested in his extensive and integrative work on biopsychological origins of affect regulation that the affective attunement between caregiver and child creates neurobiologically mediated emotional response patterns. In other words, the early interactions between infant and caretaker form a neurobiological predispositional pattern for excitement and inhibition (excitatory and inhibitory mechanisms), which constitutes a characterological feature that becomes activated in stressful situations. This is especially significant for the development of NPD and borderline personality disorder (BPD) with permanent impairments and long-term recurrent patterns of disordered mood, affect regulation, and interpersonal relationships. Schore also suggested that the patient with either NPD or BPD does not have "access to symbolic representation that can perform the important self-soothing, reparative functions encoded in evocative memory. They can not execute a reciprocal mode of autonomic control," and "their ability to autoregulate affect are fundamentally impaired" (p. 429). Schore believed that NPD and BPD represent different patterns of misattunements that contribute to their different characterological functioning.

Based on reviews of studies of attachment patterns, Schore (1994) identified two types of caregiver–child patterns that may lead to the development of NPD. An "insecure-resistant" attachment contributes to a state of hyperactivation and affect underregulation, resulting in overt grandiosity, entitlement, and aggressive reactions to others. A "depressed-hypoarousing" attachment contributes to low energy and affect overregulation, leading to inhibition, shyness, predominant shame, and hidden grandiose strivings (pp. 426–427). More specifically, in a normal grandiose positive high state of arousal, the pre-NPD child mirrors the caregiver's narcissism, and the caregiver is emotionally accessible but does not actively modulate this positive high state of arousal.

When the child is in a negative high state of arousal (e.g., aggressive separation protest), the caregiver fails to modulate the child or can even overstimulate the child into a state of dyscontrol. When the child is in a low-arousal shame/depressed state, the caregiver can not attune either to himself or herself or to the child to help the child out of this state. Overall, the caregiver is ineffective in regulating the child out of a low-arousal shame state and in offering limit setting in high-arousal states. As a result, the pre-NPD child does not develop the autonomic control and ability to neutralize grandiosity, regulate excitement, and modulate narcissistic distress.

Affect Regulation and Mentalization

Positioning themselves in the early interface between gene and environment, Fonagy, Gergely, Jurist, and Target (2002) claim that "nature (genetics and genes) operates as a 'potentialist' rather than as a 'determinist'" (p. 6). They suggest that "it is the manner in which the environment is *experienced* that acts as a filter in the expression of genotype into phenotype," and "it is the interpretation of the social environment rather than the physical environment that governs genetic expression" (p. 7). In an expanded understanding of the early development and role of mentalization as the core of this interpretation process, they highlight the function of parental affect mirroring and mental representation. They also suggest that the parents' mirroring of their child's affects helps the child to begin to reflect and realize that his or her feelings and inner experiences are separate from the outside world.

Of importance for the development of pathological narcissism and NPD is the specific mirroring structure that Fonagy and colleagues assume can predispose to NPD:

> When affect mirroring is appropriately marked but is noncontingent, in that the infant's emotion is misperceived by the caregiver, the baby will still feel the mirrored affect display to map onto his primary emotion state. However, as this mirrored state is incongruent with the infant's actual feelings, the secondary representation created will be distorted. The infant will mislabel the primary, constitutional emotional state. The self-representation will not have strong ties to the underlying emotional state. The individual

may convey an impression of reality, but as the constitutional state has not been recognized by the caregiver, the self will feel empty because it reflects the activation of secondary representations of affects that lack the corresponding connections within the constitutional self. Only when psychotherapy generates mentalized affectivity will this fault line in the psychological self be bridged." (Fonagy et al., 2002, pp. 10 – 11)

Both Schore's and Fonagy and colleagues' theoretical accounts are most useful in further explaining the internal developmental consequences of what in the previous literature has been described as the insensitivity of the parents of the "narcissist-to-become" to their child's feelings: their tendencies to assign roles and expectations to the child, to misread the child's feelings and reactions, and to ascribe their own feelings, intentions, and ambitions to their child. The child is intensively attended to and specially valued as a regulator of the parents' self-esteem, but the child is not valued and seen in his or her own right. Fonagy and colleagues (2002) noted that "the infant is forced to internalize the representation of the object's state of mind as a core part of himself" (p. 11).

Case vignette

Ms. B, an observant and very articulate woman, described her interaction with her mother the following way: "My mother could not tolerate that I had feelings. If I got upset, frightened, fuzzy, cried, or felt angry, my mother got so extremely anxious that all my attention had to focus on her and on efforts to appease her. I learned to go to my room and punch my pillow when I was sad or angry. I never learned to 'be in my own feeling' or even to know what I was feeling or how to use them. For some reason, my feelings always ended up being about my mother's feelings. Nevertheless, I learned to be the perfect daughter and not to show or even feel feelings that would upset my mother. I also learned that by being perfect I could please and control my mother. It made me feel strong and superior, and sometimes I felt that my mother was pathetic and naive, and I despised her. But underneath I was always afraid that I would lose her, that she would die and leave me."

Narcissism and Attachment

Attachment theory and classification have only recently been more systematically applied to personality disorders in general and to narcissism and NPD specifically. M. Balint's (1959) observation of defenses in the child's management of anxiety, one being to dislike attachment to others but to love the spaces between them (the philobathic attitude) is, according to Fonagy (2001), "perhaps the clearest statement of the match between analytic accounts of narcissism and a detached-dismissing attachment pattern" (p. 96). E. Balint suggested that instead of investing in objects, the child is displacing parts of his or her libido "on to the distance in space and time on the one hand, and on his developing skills on the other" (in M. Balint, 1959, p. 131). The individual learns to avoid direct satisfaction as well as dissatisfaction in interaction with others but finds satisfaction in his or her own space and activities.

Case vignette

A woman in her mid thirties was born 9 months after a sibling died in early infancy. Most of her life she had felt that she was a replacement and a substitute for her parents' loss: "I have always felt like an outsider, as if there is no real space or purpose for me. I also always sensed that I screwed up, caused problems, and aggravated people." As a child she felt best when she was alone, in her room or away from home on long walks in the forest, and she took pride in being independent and oppositional and not letting herself be influenced by other people. As an adult she noticed that she preferred to keep a distance to others by secretly mocking and criticizing them, something that added to an inner sense of superiority and satisfaction.

Another connection is Rosenfeld's (1964, 1971) model of narcissism, according to which the narcissistic individual denies the identity and separateness of another person. Fonagy (2001) suggests that Rosenfeld's "thin-skinned" narcissist matches the angry, resentful subcategory of the preoccupied adult attachment pattern, that is, being vulnerable to and confused by others, with accompanying feelings of helplessness and defectiveness that are warded off by anger. The "thick-skinned" narcissist, on the other hand, matches the dismissing pattern of attachment, that is, dumping his or her own inadequacies onto others and dismissing or devaluating the importance and influence of those people (Fonagy, 2001). Studies have rendered support for dismissing attachment in narcissistic people. Adolescents showing a dismissing attachment organization were more likely to have NPD or narcissistic traits (Rosenstein & Horowitz, 1996), and attachment avoidance was negatively related to empathy and seems to prevent access to memories of empathy (Mikulincer et al., 2001). Other studies that support the dismissing attachment pattern in narcissistic individuals refer specifically to their resistance to treatment. In order to protect themselves from the possibility that the caretaker may be unavailable, they deny their need for help (Fonagy, 2001).

Developmental Copying

A relatively new approach to understanding the vicissitudes between normal and pathological narcissism in childhood is to identify the child's coping abilities to manage the different steps in the development of narcissistic self-regulation. Such self-regulatory tasks involve gaining a sense of mastery and control, managing narcissistic vulnerability, and handling closeness, distance, and disruptions in relationships. Children approach each situation with their specific individual endowment of both healthy and pathological narcissistic functioning, and find their own solution to each task that involves both unrealistic illusions and realistic appraisals of narcissistic competence and vulnerability. In other words, it is not just the impact of a specific situation, interaction, or event that sets the stage for the development of narcissistic functioning. It is the child's own experiences and internal representations of the event, and capacity to sufficiently mentalize, self-regulate, and realistically self-assess that are crucial for the development of vicissitudes between healthy, exceptional, and pathological narcissism.

In a thoughtful and integrative article, Bleiberg (1994) suggested that "various aspects of pathological development may occur independently or may build on each other to lead to the narcissistic disorder" (p. 45). Different types of narcissistic organizations of experiences lead to subtypes of narcissistic pathology. The vulnerable child uses self-numbing, fantasized omnipotent control, and projection of intolerable self-experiences onto others to cope with circumstances that preclude normal dependency and trust. The special child with innate talents or unusual beauty or intelligence who easily evokes parents' hopes and aspirations is consequently at risk for taking on a role in the parents' self-esteem regulation. The victimized child, who experiences pain as a precondition for interpersonal relations, secretly hides a conviction of power, control, and superiority and uses pain or self-victimization to adapt and extort power (Bleiberg, 1994).

Narcissistic Parenting

Although there have been strong arguments for the critical role of narcissistic parent–child interaction and of parental projection and projective identification as an incentive to grandiosity in children, it is also evident that children of narcissistic parents do not necessarily develop narcissistic disorders. In addition, parents who contribute to the development of pathological narcissism in children or adults may not be narcissistic themselves (Elkind, 1991).

P. Kernberg (1989) made the following point: "[A]s long as the child remains outside of the parent's internal representational world, there is significantly less risk for the development of narcissistic personality disorder. Conversely, if the parent's primitive projective mechanisms involve the child excessively in the parent's own narcissistic pathology, the child is likely to also develop a narcissistic disorder" (p. 684). Modell (1975, 1980, 1991) noted that the child who accurately perceives his or her parents' intrusive, unacceptable, or unreliable behavior, because of mental disorder or eccentric reality orientation, tends to develop a premature and fragile sense of autonomy supported by omnipotence and grandiose fantasies. This "private self" can be life preserving and help the child protect a sense of separateness and ability to think for himself or herself. According to Modell (1975), this is the origin of the narcissistic defense against affects.

The first effort to systematically document observed patterns of parent–child interactions and perceptions that relate to narcissistic disorders in children and adolescents was by Rinsley (1980). Based on a self-psychological view, he identified patterns of "depersonification" where the child is being misperceived as a parental surrogate, a spouse, a sibling, or an endlessly infantile or dependent baby. The narcissistic maternal double-binding "message" is, "You may go through the motions of separating from me and appear accomplished and successful, but only if everything you achieve is ultimately in relation to me" (Rinsley, 1989, p. 702). According to Rinsley, this promotes a high degree of individuation but also a separation failure, leading to a pathological "adultomorphization." Elkind (1991) introduced the concept of "instrumental narcissism," referring to some parents' tendencies to see children as narcissistic investments whom they through their own efforts can form and make into a masterpiece, that is, a prodigy or a genius.

Parental overgratification has been considered another etiological cause of pathological narcissism. Lack of appropriate limits and feedback combined with direct or indirect evidence of being special, idealized, or overly admired makes reality attributes secondary and paves the way for grandiosity and entitlement in a child. In addition, lack of normal and optimal challenging and frustrating experiences and boundaries, as well as lack of normal disappointments, does interfere with the development of both realistic self-appraisal and self-esteem regulation, as well as with normal maturation and integration of superego (Fernando, 1998; Imbesi, 2000). Fernando (1998) identified a specific parental transference when the parent sees the child as an idealized or hated other significant (e.g., parent or sibling) from the parent's own life. The child may identify with the parent's hated relationships and intolerable self-images, and by doing so the child takes on a special role for the parent. This can lead to the parent's selective idealization of the child at the same time as it tends to undermine the parenting capability. Parents who tend to be insecure about or even abdicate their own authority and who tend to be submissive and idealize certain aspects of their child's behavior or attitudes may in a less obvious way contribute to the child's narcissistic behavior, such as entitlement, deceitfulness, and blaming, and to allow the child to control one or both parents or even the whole family.

The mother's role in the development of narcissistic character pathology has been specifically noticed in the context of boys' Oedipal strivings. In fact, experiences related to the victory of actively winning the mother or being passively seduced by her involve both omnipotent grandiosity and entitlement and the fear of retaliation from the father. Rothstein (1979, 1980) noticed that mothers who chose to overvalue and seduce their son to compensate for their husbands' failures treat such a son as a narcissistic object. In other words, the boy is assigned an omnipotent grandiose role in which he is expected to undo the humiliation caused by the devalued father/husband. Nevertheless, he is also inevitably facing a developmental defeat stemming from fear of both the father's retaliation and the mother's demands. In addition, the blurred Oedipal boundaries tend to bias the child's experiences of reality and foster an unrealistic self-image and self-appraisal in the child. Gabbard and Twemlow (1994) concluded that when such a relation becomes incestuous, it "appears to be one pathogenic pathway to the development of a hypervigilant subtype of narcissistic personality disorder" (p. 187). However, of significant importance is also both the father's response to the incestuous relationship and the overall and nonsexual nature of the mother–son relationship.

The concept of the "evil mother," repeatedly portrayed in stories with Cinderella and Snow White themes, and the mother who competes with, steals from, or otherwise controls her child's independent growth out of envy and frantic needs to possess, constitutes another type of developmental narcissistic challenge for the child (Charles, 2001).

Case vignette

A woman who just began to realize the disadvantages of her active involvement in a life long competition with her mother said: "People, including my father and brothers, always told me that I was never going to become as attractive and intelligent as my mother. Although I was convinced that they were right, they somehow spurred my urges to compete with her. But deep inside, I continued to believe that I don't deserve a good life, and that beauty, knowledge, and competence are not for me. When I met a man, I used to dread introducing him to my mother out of fear that she would seduce him and take him away from me. I notice how I have been holding on to this competition with my mother; it is as if it is the only connection I can have with her. If I resolve it, I think I will lose her."

Later in psychotherapy, this woman also discovered that an underlying stubborn defiant and rebellious attitude toward both the mother and the deceased father further added to her resistance to change and moving on in her life.

Loss of one or both parents contributes to specific intrapsychic consequences that can be relevant for development of narcissistic pathology. Rothstein (1980) considered this a trauma that the child is ill-equipped to deal with, especially due to an inability to mourn, and P. Kernberg (1989) suggested that such an experience leads to the development of a grandiose self. Fantasies involving the lost parent(s), such as heroic ideas of bringing them back, reunite with them, or being rescued by them upon their return, as well as shame for being abandoned, and unresolved guilt for having in one or another way contributed to or even caused their death (Karlsson, 1977), can in various ways affect on the development of self-esteem and affect regulation.

Childhood and Adolescent Family Roles

Berkowitz, Shapiro, Zinner, and Shapiro (1974b) noted that the family system of narcissistic adolescents exhibits certain dynamics around parents' expectations and role attributions. "In these families the child has a basic function maintaining parental self-esteem by colluding in re-enacting with the parents significant relationship that affected the parent's self-esteem in their families of origin" (p. 361). The adolescent's normal efforts to separate are perceived by the parents as a narcissistic injury and a threat to their self-esteem, and the parents react with devaluation and rage toward their adolescent's strivings for independence. Berkowitz, Shapiro, Zinner, and Shapiro (1974b) also noted the child's efforts to accommodate himself or herself to the parents' projected roles and expectations. The specific omnipotent power involved in being able to influence the parents' self-experiences and self-esteem is both seductive and narcissistically gratifying for the child. It also increases the child's or adolescent's reluctance to move on with his or her own independent life tasks because separation may trigger fear of the parents' rage and abandonment.

Case vignette

A young woman, who lived with her parents after having failed in her efforts to make a career as a musician, said: "I am convinced that my parents' marriage will fall apart and that we will never speak to each other again if I move on in my life. I feel as if I have been the uniting force in my parents' life and maybe even in my extensive family. I am the oldest and I was supposed to make it. Both my great grandmother, my grandmother, and my three aunts died of breast cancer when I was a child. My mother was terrified, she turned to me and I became in a peculiar way her evidence of life, her motivation and reason to stay alive and continue and live with my father. I felt as if I was the strongest."

Although both parents in this family had lived an active and productive life, the perceived psychological meaning of the parents' grief, fear, and expectations had apparently assumed a narcissistic function and meaning in this woman when she was a child.

P. Kernberg (1989, 1998) identified several roles or functions that are beyond or inconsistent with the child's normal and age-appropriate developmental tasks. An example of such a role is the child of a single parent who takes on the omnipotent task of replacing the missing parent.

Case vignette

A gay man in his mid forties said, "When I was 8 years old my father left the family, and I became my mother's confidant. My mother did not understand men. She made a lot of efforts to meet a new man in her life, but she had difficulties. I used to tell her what to do, and when looking back I actually believe I gave her exceptionally good advice, but for some reason she always screwed up. As a teenager I went dancing with my mother to make sure she chose men who were good for her. She was a very charming and strikingly attractive woman. I never felt I had a mother, more a friend. We are actually still friends, although I have never been able to confide in her when I have problems with my partners, for example; she is too preoccupied with herself."

Another role is the adopted child who has experienced being both chosen by the adoptive parents and abandoned by the biological parents. In other words, such a child struggles with an inner sense of being both special and chosen, and "nonspecial" and "nonchosen." The abused child, on the other hand, merges with an idealized image of the abusing parent to protect himself or herself from the sadistic image of the abuser and from the experience of being abused (P. Kernberg, 1989, 1998).

Case vignette

A woman in her mid fifties tended to marginalize the influence of her father, whom she described as naive, harmless, low class, and not specifically intelligent. She compared him to her grandfather, who had adored her and considered her to be his special granddaughter, and to her husband, whom she saw as the total opposite to her father—smart, influential, upper class, and very considerate. After several months in psychotherapy, she referred to her father's explosive rage outbursts and described feeling horrified, helpless, and physically overwhelmed when watching her father verbally and physically attacking her two older sisters. She had deliberately chosen to cope with her father's rage by behaving totally opposite to her sisters, that is, by being a perfect, quiet, obedient daughter and an excellent student. She felt protected because she believed that by avoiding her sisters' provocative and oppositional behavior, which ultimately evoked the father's rage, she could control her father, the abuser. On the other hand, as an adult she noticed that when she got angry she felt as if she became her father, and she had difficulties differentiating the experiences of her own anger from the anger of her father.

The child of narcissistic parents, who is indulged and has special expectations assigned, tends to develop a strong sense of entitlement and omnipotent control, infantile narcissism, and grandiosity, later combined with frustration and anger.

Case vignette

After having made a serious suicide attempt, a young man said, "My parents have high expectations for me—I am the one, actually the only one in my entire family who can become a medical doctor. They have always given me everything I ever wanted, but they also always had only one thing in the back of their mind—they wanted me to become a doctor!!!"

T: "How do you feel about that now?"
P: "I actually feel desperate. I used to feel great about it, but last week I began to feel that I don't have any choices. I am terrified of disappointing my family. I don't even know if I want to go to medical school. I do know that I want to surpass my stupid cousins and my unbearable brother, because I know I am very smart. But what if I fail? Right now, a career as a medical doctor appears like an unbearable chore. I can't even stand the thought of it."

Conclusions on the Origins of NPD

This brief review indicates several avenues that may lead to the development of pathological narcissism. It also indicates that pathological narcissism has both genetic and early developmental origins but may still be less obvious in childhood and become more overtly noticeable in adulthood when the individual is facing other and more narcissistically challenging life tasks. So far, our understanding of the early origins of pathological narcissism leans on theoretical inferences and clinical observations that yet await empirical verifications. The interface between psychoanalytic and academic psychological observations of early infants and parent–child interactions, and of patterns in family systems offers many possibilities for future research that can explore and identify the specific and crucial etiological conditions for pathological narcissism.

The Scope of Narcissistic Personality Disorder

How Common Is NPD?

Although there is a general sense that narcissistic disorders are becoming more common in Western society, the prevalence rate of NPD in the general population is still very low (0–0.4%), suggesting that NPD is among the least common personality disorders (Mattia & Zimmerman, 2001). Others report consistent low to moderate prevalence rates, less than 1% in the general population (J. Reich, Yates, & Ndvaguba, 1989;Torgersen, Kringlen, & Cramer, 2001). A few studies have found somewhat higher rates of NPD, 3.9–5.3% (Bodlund, Ekselius, & Lindström, 1993; D. N. Klein et al., 1995) using nonclinical control samples. Studies also indicate that NPD is more frequently found among people in higher education or special professional groups. In a study of personality maladjustment among first-year medical students, 17% met criteria for NPD (Maffei et al., 1995), and narcissistic personality traits or NPD was the most commonly occurring Axis II diagnosis (20%) in a military clinical outpatient sample (Bourgeois, Crosby, Hall, Drexler, 1993; Crosby & Hall, 1992). W. Johnson (1995) suggested that military service may appeal to narcissistic people because of the focus on appearance, rewards, and public displays of reinforcement.

The use of the NPD diagnosis is probably more common in some clinical settings such as forensic psychiatric clinics and private hospitals or in the private practices of psychoanalysts, psychotherapists, and marriage counselors. In the adult clinical population, rates between 2% and 16% have been found (Gunderson, Ronningstam, & Smith, 1991), and high rates of NPD were identified in the personality disorder population (22%; Morey 1988) as well as in specific clinical samples. A study of cocaine abusers reported that 32% had a comorbid diagnosis of NPD (Yates, Fulton, Gabel, & Brass, 1989). In a sample of bipolar patients, 47% met criteria for NPD (Turley, Bates, Edwards, & Jackson, 1992), and in a Japanese study on personality disorders in depression (Sato et al., 1997), 21% met the *DSM-III-R* diagnostic criteria for NPD. Studies of prevalence in clinical populations do not reflect clinicians' usage of the NPD diagnosis, and the *DSM* criteria often fail to identify patients whom clinicians consider having a NPD diagnosis. Only 10 of 24 patients clinically diagnosed as NPD met the threshold for the *DSM-III-R* NPD diagnosis (Gunderson et al., 1991).

Most prevalence studies have used diagnostic interviews or questionnaires to identify narcissistic patients. The variations in cultural expressions, clinical presentation, and level of functioning in people with narcissistic disorders contribute to a significant difficulty in establishing consistent prevalence rates using brief and structured diagnostic measures. Some people with NPD present themselves as obliviously arrogant, boastful, attention seeking, and entitled, and they bluntly and even proudly verify their narcissistic characteristics. Others may pride themselves on being modest and secretly but consciously hide their narcissistic strivings, or they may, due to shame and insecurity, deny any tendencies of feeling special or superior or of having serious interpersonal problems. Because they appear sensitive, compliant, timid, and suffering from feelings of inferiority, an extended psychodiagnostic evaluation or a longer period of psychotherapy may be required to establish a correct diagnosis. Still other narcissistic people who present closer to the psychopathy range are ruthlessly insensitive and entitledly exploitative, charming, and cunning with manipulative and sadistic behavior (Harpur, Hare, & Hakstian, 1989; O. Kernberg, 1998). In addition, of diagnostic and clinical importance is the fact that people who initially may present strikingly overt narcissistic features can paradoxically have less severe narcissistic pathology and be capable of both empathy and interpersonal commitments. Others who appear concerned and interpersonally "tuned in" can have a much more severe hidden underlying narcissistic pathology, being cunning, envious, spiteful, contemptuous, revengeful, and incapable of mutual interpersonal relationships. In sum, there are significant ambiguities in differentiating narcissistic traits from the enduring NPD, and in the absence of relevant definitions and cutoff points for NPD, the use of the terms is relatively arbitrary. In other words, people can have specific areas of severely disordered narcissism without meeting the criteria for NPD, and people can also have severe NPD without meeting the official criteria. None of the present diagnostic systems or instruments takes into account these diagnostic challenges.

Male or Female Disorder?

Research reports disagree on the gender distribution of NPD. Some studies support the idea that NPD is more common in males than in females (Golomb et al., 1995; Ronningstam & Gunderson, 1990; Torgersen et al., 2001), while others believe NPD is equally prevalent in both sexes (Plakun, 1990). *DSM-IV* claims that 50–75% of those diagnosed with NPD are male. Ninety-five percent of patients diagnosed as narcissistic (with traits or personality disorder) in a military sample were male, indicating a professionally related gender difference (Crosby & Hall, 1992).

One study of gender differences found that men and women express narcissistic issues in different ways (Reichman & Flaherty, 1990), and the authors claimed that the present conceptualization of narcissism reflects a predominantly male expression of the disorder. Men manifest a greater sense of uniqueness, more interpersonal exploitativeness, entitlement and lack of empathy, while women show more intense reactiveness to slights from others (Reichman & Flaherty, 1990). Recognition of covert narcissistic characteristics may also help identify specific narcissistic patterns in women.

Age Differences

Narcissistic disturbances are frequent among people in their late teens and early twenties, due to the specific developmental challenges in the transition from adolescence to adulthood. Such disturbances are usually corrected through developmental life experiences and normally do not develop into adult NPD (Ronningstam, Gunderson, & Lyons, 1995). However, the presence of NPD in both children and adolescents has been empirically verified (Abrams, 1993; P. Kernberg, Hajal, & Normandin, 1998). P. Kernberg (1989, 1998) noted that the narcissistic features found in adults also may be seen in children, that is, excessive demandingness, omnipotent control, self-absorption, grandiose fantasies, possessiveness, and lack of empathy. Narcissistic children also have a checkered performance in school and poor peer interactions. They show gaze aversion to protect their grandiosity, avoid depersonification from narcissistically possessive parents, and disavow dependency on other people. They also show separation anxiety underneath a surface of self-sufficiency.

Unlike other dramatic cluster disorders, NPD does not necessarily remit with advanced age. In fact, middle age is an especially critical period for the development or worsening of NPD. The challenge of facing such personal and professional limitations as lost opportunities, loss of parents, and increased independence of their children can reinforce specific pathological or defensive narcissistic traits, leading to chronic denial, emptiness, devaluation, guilt, and cynicism (O. F. Kernberg, 1980). Significant narcissistic pathology and personality disorder have also been found in elderly people (Berezin, 1977; O. Kernberg, 1977). In addition, normal changes in old age such as facing retirement, declined physical health attraction and strength, and other expected changes and losses can also reveal lifelong narcissistic imbalances and accompanying regrets, resentment, self-accusations and grief.

Case vignette

Ms D had been an executive secretary in a very exclusive and financially secure company for 37 years and served two consecutive presidents. She had over the years been immensely appreciated for her hard work and extraordinary administrative knowledge and capacity, and adored for her refined and cultivated personal manners. Indeed, she had been the president's right hand and assigned as the top cognizant of the company's present whereabouts as well as its history. She was the natural participant both at their business and family events. She had a spotless work record and had been considered the perfect indispensable secretary. Reaching 65, she was facing retirement and the company arranged a festive and generous goodbye party for her at which she received huge recognition and substantial retirement benefits. A few months later Ms D got severely depressed and was referred to psychotherapy by her physician. Uncomfortable in this new situation as a recipient of help and having to reveal her personal history beyond her extraordinary professional life, she nevertheless confided in her therapist and told the following story. After her graduation, the parents suddenly got quite ill and they both imposed upon Ms D to take care of her mentally retarded sister, 3 years older, who had never lived outside the parents' home. Ms D described feeling torn between obligation and grief toward the parents who both died shortly after, and overwhelming and painful pity and resentment toward her severely handicapped sister. At that time she was offered the job as executive secretary and Ms D felt that she entered something of a heaven, with an opportunity to work for an extraordinary man in an exclusive company. Throughout her adult life she remained unmarried, continued to live in her deceased parents' home, and remained loyal to both her sister and her presidents. After retirement she was facing a severe sense of loss, emptiness, and loneliness. She was overwhelmed by regrets for not having been married, for not having had the courage to initiate changes in her burdensome commitment vis-à-vis her sister, and for not having pursued her initial dream of going to medical school and having a professional career of her own. Psychotherapy helped this woman to some degree to understand and accept her choices in life and to grieve lost opportunities.

Conclusion on the Scope of NPD

The traditional notion that disordered narcissism is mainly an adult male phenomenon has been challenged by numerous studies that have shown that narcissistic self-esteem and affect dysregulation do occur throughout the lifespan from childhood to old age. Although the diagnosis of NPD may be more often given to men, especially when including violent and psychopathic behavior, other features and expressions of pathological narcissism, that is, the more subtle and internally hidden, seem more predominant in women. Future studies of narcissistic gender variations and variations in male and female self-esteem regulation are welcome.

Narcissistic Personalities in the Movies

Several narcissistic personalities have over the years been well characterized in films. Most of them have been striking and easily identified as the typical arrogant or psychopathic narcissistic type, such as Michael Caine's portrayal of Graham Marshall in *Shock to the System*, Charles Boyer's portrayal of Gregory Anton in *Gaslight*, and Roy Scheider's portrayal of Joseph Gideon (a.k.a. Bob Fosse) in *All That Jazz*. Two recent French films, however, *Read My Lips*, by Jacques Audiard, staring Emmanuelle Devos and Vincent Cassel, and *The Piano Teacher*, by Michael Haneke (from a novel by Elfride Jelinek) starring Isabelle Huppert and Benoit Magimel, beautifully portray the shy and more discreetly presented but still severely disturbed narcissistic personality. Carla Bhem (actress Emmanuelle Devos in *Read My Lips*), a lonely, hearing-impaired, stress-sensitive, underpaid, and badly treated office manager with an exceptional capacity to read lips, surprises the audience with her interpersonal control, personal impact, and capacity for vengefulness. Erika Kohut (in *The Piano Teacher*, played by Isabelle Huppert), a sensitive but stoic and perfectionist music professor and pianist, shows amazing cruelty and sadomasochistic demeanor toward her students as the piano teacher and toward her intrusive and controlling mother with whom she lives and shares a bedroom. We follow the encounters between these women and their male partners—Paul, an unskilled office aid just released from jail, and Walter, an exceptionally handsome and gifted piano student. While Carla and Erika both initially resist and then quickly gain dominance over their partners' sexual advances, they also have vivid fantasies about their own sexual roles and experiences in such encounters. Carla's seemingly erratic and submissive behavior is, nevertheless, accompanied by a remarkable capacity for recollection, cooperation, and enjoyment of triumph that gradually develops to intimacy and her involvement in passionate intercourse with Paul after a joint successful criminal endeavor. However, Erika's refined manners and calculating presence cover a deep confusion and repulsion toward intimacy. As her dominance is subverted, she becomes increasingly desperate, and Walter's attempts to pursue his own desire as he tries to read and fulfill her sadistic instructions lead to Erika's personal disintegration and ultimate detachment.

Conclusion

This chapter has discussed the two most essential features that give sufficient grounds for justifying pathological narcissism as a disorder, that is, its genetic and developmental origins and its prevalence in different communities, settings and population groups. Research on early development of affect regulation and empathic capacity is especially important for identifying the vulnerability for self-esteem dysregulation and pathological narcissism. Narcissistic disorders and NPD are not easily identifiable with diagnostic instruments used in epidemiological studies and people with disordered narcissism tend to be relatively high functioning and usually not found in psychiatric settings. This has contributed to a discrepancy between narcissism representing a rare personality disorder to the common notion that narcissistic behavior has become increasingly common in the Western world.

4

Identifying Pathological Narcissism

The terms "pathological narcissism," "narcissistic disorder," and "narcissistic personality disorder" (NPD) have often been used interchangeably in the clinical literature. Other terms such as "narcissistic" and narcissistic "disturbances," "features," and "traits" also frequently occur in both clinical and social psychological discussions, often without any further definition. This chapter outlines and describes strategies for identifying pathological narcissism and NPD in terms of self-esteem and affect regulation, interpersonal relativeness, and superego functioning, as well as the clinical presentation of some of the significant narcissistic characteristics. For the purposes of clarity, the following definitions of pathological narcissism, narcissistic traits/features/characteristics, narcissistic disorder, and NPD will be used throughout this volume.

Pathological narcissism differs from healthy or normal narcissism because self-esteem is dysregulated, serving to protect and support a grandiose but fragile self. Affect regulation is compromised by difficulties in processing and modulating feelings, specifically anger, shame, and envy. Interpersonal relationships are also affected because they are used primarily to protect or enhance the self-esteem and other self-regulatory functions at the expense of mutual relativeness and intimacy. This definition refers to narcissism as a dimension ranging from healthy to pathological and to the long-term NPD. Pathological narcissism is identified by degree of severity, dominance of aggression versus shame, and by the extent to which its manifestations are overt or covert.

Pathological narcissism can be more or less obtrusive on an individual's sustained personality functioning. When the level of pathological narcissism is less severe, temporary, situational, or limited to a set of specific character features that interfere to a lesser degree with regular personal, interpersonal, and/or vocational functioning, it is referred to as "narcissistic disturbance," "disordered narcissism," or "narcissistic traits." The diagnostic term "narcissistic personality disorder" refers to a stable long-term characterological functioning that meets the criteria for NPD in the *DSM-IV* or any other comprehensive diagnostic description of this character disorder, including the covert, shy type (Akhtar, 1989, 1997; Cooper, 1998; Cooper & Ronningstam, 1992; Gabbard, 1989; O. Kernberg, 1983, 1985; Ronningstam & Gunderson, 1990). NPD refers to specific deformations in the personality structure that involve a pathological grandiose self, leading to problems in self-regulation. The self-esteem is inconsistent, fragile, and maintained by pathologically defensive, expressive, and supportive regulatory processes. Affect regulation is influenced by feelings of rage, shame, and envy, and the capacity for empathy and interpersonal commitment is impaired. Superego functioning is also inconsistent and/or overly harsh.

In addition, in a recently proposed diagnostic term, "trauma-associated narcissistic symptoms" (Simon, 2001), the stress associated with an external traumatic experience overwhelm the self and trigger symptoms such as shame, humiliation, and rage. Although underlying vulnerability to such stress can stem from the presence of pathological narcissism or NPD, even people with relatively healthy self-esteem can develop narcissistic symptoms after experiencing a more or less severe narcissistic humiliation.

These definitions indicate the complexity of pathological narcissism, that is, that there are context-dependent, reactive types of pathological narcissism with changeability and fluctuations between healthy and pathological narcissistic functioning, as well as more enduring, stable forms of NPD with clearly identifiable character pathology and a long-term course (Ronningstam, Gunderson, & Lyons, 1995). These definitions also suggest that pathological narcissism encompasses different levels of functioning or degrees of severity. They can range from extraordinarily high levels of functioning combined with exceptional capabilities, to context-determined narcissistic reactions, to a personality disorder with mild to severe limitations and disabled functioning in interpersonal and vocational areas, to malignant forms of narcissism and antisocial or psychopathic behavior found in severe criminals (Groopman & Cooper, 1995; O. Kernberg, 1998a). Pathological narcissism can, independent of level of severity, range from being overt, striking, and obtrusive to being internally concealed and unnoticeable. Furthermore, pathological narcissism can also appear together with other forms of character pathology or major mental disorders and interact with other significant personality characteristics or symptomatology such as psychopathy, borderline personality disorder (BPD), the bipolar spectrum disorder, eating disorders, and others. Vicissitudes between healthy and more or less severe pathological narcissism are constantly present, and the coexistence of and intertwined interaction between healthy and pathological aspects of narcissistic functioning can make it specifically challenging to identify and understand the narcissistic personality (Kohut, 1966; Watson & Biderman, 1993).

This complexity of narcissism might prompt the reader to ask how it is possible that pathological narcissism can encompass all these varieties of symptoms and levels of functioning, and whether NPD really is just one disorder. The purpose of this chapter is to address these discrepancies and divergences along a dimensional model for narcissism that can encompass and explain the range of clinical expressions from healthy and constructive narcissism to the extreme pathological forms (see table 4.1). This model ranges from healthy and exceptional narcissism to pathological traits, to the enduring NPD, and it includes the shy, the arrogant, and the psychopathic types of NPD. This model also takes into account the degree of severity, dominance of aggression versus shame, and extent to which its manifestations are overt or internally hidden. In addition, this model accounts for the vicissitudes between healthy and pathological forms of narcissism.

Narcissistic Traits

The presence of one or a few narcissistic traits may easily be overlooked or remain unidentified, especially if the person is generally well functioning or has other more obvious signs of psychopathology. Narcissistic traits can be more or less overt and intrusive and be experienced as more or less handicapping to the individual's functioning. For example, a skilled anesthesiologist is less likely to experience problems when exhibiting arrogant behavior in his professional career, whereas for somebody applying for a position as an elementary school teacher or a nurse, arrogant behavior may be considered an obstacle. Likewise, people with certain narcissistic traits may appear more strikingly offensive, such as those with aggres-

Table 4.1. The range of narcissism from healthy and extraordinary to the types of narcissistic personality disorders.

Dimensions of narcissism	Healthy narcissism	Extraordinary narcissism	Pathological narcissism		
			Arrogant	Shy	Psychopathic
Self-esteem regulation	Realistic self-appraisal of both abilities and limitations; capacity to tolerate disapproval, criticism and rejection as well as realistic approval and praise of real accomplishments and successes. Grandiose fantasies function as motivators and guidelines for achievements and goals.	Heightened self-confidence and self-worth, sense of self-invulnerability. Capacity for unusual risk taking and decision making, and to integrate unusual ideas, ideals and goals into real achievements or creative accomplishments	Inflated and vulnerable self-esteem with inner sense of superiority and uniqueness, Strong reactions to criticism, defeats or other threats to the self-esteem. Grandiose fantasies support and enhance self-esteem	Inhibitions prevents actual self-appraisal and development of real capability. Shame for ambitions and grandiose aims. Compensatory grandiose fantasies of being special or perfect; intolerance of criticism	Immoral, violent or psychopathic behavior serve to protect or enhance the inflated self experience
Affect regulation	Healthy affect regulation with ability to feel self-conscious emotions such as envy, shame and pride, and tolerance to feeling inferiority and humiliation, as well as to challenge and success-related	Exceptional capacity to feel certain feelings related to tasks or goals.	Strong feelings of anger, shame and envy; hyperreactivity to perceived humiliations and threats to self-esteem . Mood variations including depression, irritability, elation or hypomania reflect shifting levels of self-esteem.	Hypersensitivity and low affect tolerance; intense shame reactions and fear of failure. Affect inhibition and hypochondria	Extreme hyperreactivity with aggressive and violent behavior Predominance of envy and rage

	excitement; ability to internal control, sense of power and constructive aggression.				
Interpersonal relationships	Self-preservation, self-regard, and healthy entitlement involving ability to feel that one deserve what is earned or received. Ability for empathy and compassion, and a sense of belongingness and appreciation of commitment and mutual relationships	Heightened entitlement ability to feel that one deserve extraordinary circumstances or endowments, ability to take on exceptional roles and tasks. Heightened exhibitionism, potentials for leadership, charisma, and capacity to conceptualize and embody ideas or mission in relationship to others. Exceptional capacity for devotion.	Interpersonal relations serve to protect and enhance self-esteem: arrogant and haughty attitude, seeking admiring attention, and entitled and controlling and hostile behavior. Impaired empathic processing, and capacity for commitments.	Interpersonal and vocational inhibitions; low tolerance for exhibitionism and attention from others; hypersensitive to humiliation and criticism; appears attentive, modest, and humble. Impaired capacity for empathy and genuine commitments to others; strong feelings of envy	Entitled exploitativeness irritability and rage reactions; strong feelings of envy; interpersonal sadism and revengefulness.
Super-ego regulation	Super-ego regulation involving self approval, pride, constructive self-criticism, and realistic balance between attainable ideals and actual capability	Superego regulation with exceptional ideals, high and unusual standards for performance and achievement, unusual sense of responsibility and commitment to a specific task or role	Compromised or inconsistent superego functioning ranging from temporary extreme moral perfectionism to corruptive consciousness, deceitful manipulative behavior, one or a few crimes.	Higher moral standards, strict conscience, and harsh self-criticism; unattainable and hidden ideals; ability to feel remorse and guilt	Severe super-ego pathology with sadistic, malignant or antisocial behavior. Idealization of criminal or violent behavior; lack of remorse or guilt

sive entitlement or with the combination of superiority, condescending attitude, and interpersonally controlling, manipulative, and demanding behavior. Usually, such people come across as dislikable and can evoke strong negative reactions in other people. In contrast, a shy, seemingly subdued but ambitious person who is appealing and evokes sympathy and friendly feelings in others can have hidden grandiose strivings and a more serious incapacity for empathy and close relationships or tendencies to specific context-dependent rage reactions concealed underneath good social manners. Furthermore, such shy appearance may actually represent a more severe narcissistic pathology compared to the overtly offensive and dislikable one. In addition, unexpected or even normal life changes or other challenges can exacerbate narcissistic traits that reflect the individual's reactions to or way of managing such events.

Case vignette

A successful lawyer in his early fifties had over the years developed and taken pride in his unusual people skills. He was considered an exceptionally patient, understanding, and tolerant person by his clients and colleagues. Nevertheless, as his son and daughter were reaching their mid teens, he was unable to tolerate what he considered their sudden and extreme behavioral changes. He felt rejected and humiliated by their attitudes and choice of cloths, friends, and music. He felt unable to communicate with and guide them as he had done before, and he experienced this as a personal failure and defeat. He reacted strongly with irritability and rage outbursts and feelings of insecurity and shame.

The presence of pathological narcissism or narcissistic traits may be specifically important to identify when they co-occur with other psychiatric symptoms such as posttraumatic stress disorder, eating disorders, borderline personality disorder, or bipolar disorder (see chapter 5 this volume). Aspects of narcissistic self-esteem or affect regulation can involve major significant symptoms and influence the person's motivation for treatment, and consequently the treatment outcome and prognosis. In other words, a specific symptom may be important for self-esteem regulation and contribute to increased achievement or to a sense of pride or control. For example, for some patients with bipolar disorder, the positive effects of hypomania on creativity and professional productivity can be a major source of narcissistic self-esteem regulation that is lost in a euthymic phase.

Case vignette

An extremely smart and arrogant young man diagnosed with bipolar disorder had been putting off writing his master's thesis. Facing graduation, he stopped mood-stabilizing psychopharmacological treatment, entered into an elevated mood state, and began working 15–18 hours a day researching and writing. He finished his thesis in time and graduated with honors but was hospitalized shortly after in a state of acute mania. He felt proud and superior because he had done his thesis in seven weeks while his peers had spent several months finishing theirs. He took a risk, which he liked to do, and considered spending 10 days in mental hospital a small price to pay for such a "peak achievement." He liked his elevated mood or hypomania, because it increased his working capacity and made him more productive and able to multitask, that is, to work on several problems simultaneously. In addition, he noticed that his thinking became more creative, sharper, and expansive and that his self-esteem increased and he felt confident. Back in a more euthymic phase, he said: "If necessary, I would do it again."

Similarly, the experience of control of weight and body image in anorexia is often associated with a sense of superiority, well-being, and high self-esteem, which is lessened with weight gain. Impulsive self-destructive rage reactions in borderline patients who experience abandonment can at times alternate or coexist with entitled narcissistic rage reactions due to humiliated pride and feelings of indignation and degradation. Likewise, a stoic, superior, and haughty attitude may hide an underlying emotional trauma. Acknowledgment of these differences may be crucial to the patient's treatment response and progress.

Narcissistic Personality Disorder—The Arrogant Type

The official guidelines for diagnosing NPD are the criteria set and diagnostic description found in the *DSM-IV* and *DSM-IV-TR* (see the appendix to this volume). Narcissistic personalities are usually identified by overt and striking grandiosity: a sense of superiority and self-importance, a tendency to exaggerate talents or achievement, and a belief in being special and unique. Grandiose fantasies of success, power, brilliance, and so forth, serve to expand their sense of themselves. Entitlement—unreasonable expectations of especially favorable treatment—the need for excessive admiration, and arrogant and haughty behavior characterize interactions with other people. In addition, envy of others or the belief that others envy them, and unempathic and exploitative attitudes and behavior toward other people or society are additional character traits that impair the narcissistic individual's capacity for interpersonal functioning and long-term commitments (*DSM-IV, DSM-IV-TR*).

Beyond the *DSM*, there is by now both clinical and empirical support for identifying the core of narcissistic pathology as centering on four major areas of functioning: self-esteem regulation, affect regulation, interpersonal relationships, and superego functioning. In addition, several accounts support the existence of three subtypes of NPD: (1) the arrogant, oblivious, overt type; (2) the shy, hypervigilant, covert type; and (3) the psychopathic narcissistic type.

Self-esteem Regulation

Narcissism has historically been associated with self-esteem, and defects in self-esteem regulation, usually described in terms of inflated or vulnerable self-esteem, is one of the core disturbances in narcissistic disorder (Goldberg, 1973; O. Kernberg, 1975; Kohut, 1971; A. Reich, 1960). In a study of psychodynamic conflicts in narcissistic people, J. D. C. Perry and J. C. Perry (2004) concluded that most significant conflicts associated to NPD related to problems with self-esteem regulation, that is, rejection of others, ambition achievement, dominant goals, resentment over being thwarted by others, and counterdependence. An outstanding feature of narcissistic peoples' self-esteem is the instability. Recent research (Kernis, Cornell, Sun, Berry, & Harlow, 1993) has found that people with unstable self-esteem have more fluctuations in self-evaluation and place greater importance on such self-evaluations for determining their overall self-worth. Rhodewalt and colleagues (Rhodewalt, Madrian, & Cheney, 1998; Rhodewalt & Morf, 1998) concluded that narcissistic people have greater self-esteem instability and mood variability, are more sensitive to ego threats that lower their self-esteem, and tend to react with anger and hostility to such threats. Rhodewalt also suggested that self-aggrandizing and self-attributions used for protection of the grandiose self cause hypersensitivity to criticism and more extreme reactions to both success and failure. Narcissistic people externalize failure and attribute success to their own ability—a strategy that sets the stage for narcissistic rage reactions.

In the context of psychobiological self-regulatory processes, especially affect regulation, self-esteem has also been conceptualized as an "affective picture of the self," with positive affects, such as joy and excitement, related to high self-esteem and negative affects, such as shame, to low self-esteem. Schore (1994, pp. 362–365) suggests that shame, a regulator of positive and negative affects, is also a regulator of self-esteem and a modulator of success and failure in competence, of active interest and expectations, and of exploratory and stress-managing behavior. In other words, the presence of shame is associated with detachment and experiences of incompetence, while in the absence of shame the self is seeking attachment and involvement in competence-enhancing activities. Anger can also serve as a self-esteem regulator, that is, as a defensive reaction to ward off threats and avoid a lowering or loss of self-esteem. Sometimes anger can even increase self-esteem (Baumeister, Smart, & Boden, 1996; Dodes, 1990).

Captured under the umbrella of grandiosity, self-esteem dysregulation serves to maintain inflated self-experiences and undo feelings of inadequacy and insufficiency. Studies have also identified narcissism as a defensive form of self-esteem regulation (Kernis & Sun, 1994; Raskin, Novacek & Hogan, 1991). These studies verified that narcissistic self-esteem management, consisting of dominance, hostility, and grandiosity (Raskin et al., 1991), serves to enhance the vulnerable grandiose self and protect it from self-doubt and feelings of inferiority and insufficiency. In addition, it protects against other threatening feelings such as anger, anxiety, fear, shame, and depression. In other words, narcissistic individuals with an inflated self-view and high but unstable self-esteem tend to dominate and control situations and other people and react with anger and hostility toward perceived threats to their positive self-regard and self-esteem (Bushman& Baumeister 1998; Kernis, Granneman, & Barclay, 1989; Smalley & Stake, 1996). They also react with increased optimism and unrealistic goal setting, leading to impaired judgment and risk of self-regulation failure (Baumeister, Heatheron, & Tice, 1993).

Grandiosity In clinical settings, characteristics describing grandiosity differentiate narcissistic patients from all other patients (Ronningstam

& Gunderson, 1990). Grandiosity refers to an unrealistic sense of superiority, a sustained view of oneself as better than others that causes the
narcissistic person to view others with disdain or as different or inferior.
It also refers to a sense of uniqueness, the belief that few others have
much in common with oneself and that one can only be understood
by a few or very special people. Additional attitudes and behaviors that
serve to support and enhance the inflated self-esteem include admiring
attention seeking, boastful and pretentious attitudes, and unrestrained
self-centered and self-referential behavior. Grandiose fantasies serve to
protect, complement, or expand the grandiose self-experience. Narcissistic fantasies stem from a need to change the self to overcompensate
for experienced defects. The fantasies are self-directed and more experiential rather than narrative, and they focus on being different and exceptional. Among other things, such fantasies concern the self's uniqueness
and perfection and the search for transcendence of earthly limitations
(Bach, 1977a).

Grandiosity has been considered the core trait and the distinguishing characteristic differentiating NPD from both BPD and antisocial
personality disorder (ASPD). Nevertheless, grandiosity is also reactive
and state dependent (Ronningstam et al., 1995). For instance, it can be
influenced by brief depressive reactions or depressive disorder, causing
a more self-critical and humble attitude, or by moving from late adolescence to adulthood with experiences of more realistic achievements
and interpersonal experiences that stabilize the self-esteem. It can also
be influenced by corrective life events, such as achievements and disillusionments that contribute to a more realistic alignment of the self-
esteem and evaluation of one's own capacity and potential. In addition,
sudden threats to the self-esteem can temporarily increase expressions
of a defensive grandiose self-experience (Simon, 2001). Differentiating between state-dependent signs or temporary increase of grandiosity
and stable symptoms of grandiose self-experience may require specific
diagnostic attention. This changeability in grandiosity suggests that the
diagnosis of NPD should not depend as heavily on grandiosity as has
been suggested in the empirical and clinical literature (Ronningstam et
al., 1995).

Real or Exaggerated Achievements   Closely related to grandiosity is the
narcissistic individuals' tendency to make self-aggrandizing attributions
to enhance self-esteem (Rhodewalt & Morf, 1998) and exaggerate their

talents and achievements (Ronningstam & Gunderson, 1990). Many narcissistic people are indeed very capable and do have sustained periods of successful academic, professional, or creative accomplishments. The combination of exceptional talents or intellectual giftedness, grandiose fantasies, and strong self-investment can, in certain cases, lead to extraordinary intellectual, creative, or innovative contributions (see chapter 6 this volume). Such a capacity may compensate for or counterbalance other interpersonal or emotional difficulties that the narcissistic person experiences in other areas in life. Although high achievements are not considered a diagnostic criterion, their presence distinguishes people with NPD from those with most other personality disorders (Ronningstam & Gunderson, 1990). The capacity for high achievement is frequently a source or justification of a sense of superiority—a reason for the importance of doing a thorough evaluation of both unrealistic and realistic aspects of actual capability, high self-esteem, and superiority. It is specifically important to differentiate realistic competence and high self-esteem in a person coming across as haughty and superior from defensive unrealistic exaggerations and bragging, as well as from actual potentials and capabilities that may be hidden behind grandiose fantasies or an arrogant disdainful or insecure, shy attitude.

Case vignette

Mr. M, a smart but arrogant and oppositional man in his twenties, had taken pride in criticizing, ridiculing, and outsmarting teachers and peers. He engaged in self-defeating demonstrations of his high intellectual and athletic capability by sabotaging lectures and destroying relationships. Both his parents and his counselors had doubts that he would be able to pursue a career or even make a decent living given his irresponsible and uncooperative personality. However, after graduation Mr. M got a job as a squash teacher in a remotely located small college. This work gave him an opportunity to realize his athletic abilities, develop his own teaching strategies, form relationships with his students, and promote their learning and personal and athletic growth. He felt that he had an opportunity to realize his wish to be better than his own teachers. His superior critical attitude was transformed into high but realistic professional ambitions and standards, and he actually became appreciated among both his students and colleagues.

The Seemingly Opposite—Masochism and Martyr Roles   Some people may be caught in an experientially shame-filled cycle of proving themselves capable of an assigned special but impossible task and constantly fighting a sense of incompetence. Often, and paradoxically, these people may experience themselves as singled out and specially chosen but also caught in a role with special responsibilities and expectations that puts constraints and burdens on normal development and interpersonal life. The person may even be victimized, or trapped in a martyr role or in a sadomasochistic position. When suffering and victimization are associated with grandiosity and entitlement, such experiences become a means to regulate self-esteem and self-worth, as in the narcissistic-masochistic character (Cooper, 1988, 1998). Suffering is ego-syntonic, and the individual experiences a sense of mastery and control of his own humiliations. Chronic self-pity, originally a response to narcissistic humiliation or empathic failure and an attempt to counteract feelings of alienation and disintegration, is a state that involves both pain and pleasure and is often accompanied by self-righteousness and hostility (S. Wilson, 1985).

Case vignette

Mr. C's close relationship to his father was interrupted in childhood when his father unexpectedly became ill. From then on, he had struggled to regain closeness to and appreciation from his emotionally distant father. He said, "When I got accepted to one of the most prestigious graduate schools in the country I noticed how my father changed. He began to ridicule me, showed more interest in my friends than in me. He stopped talking to me for long periods, and he even threatened to stop paying my tuition."

T: "That was obviously not what you had expected."
C: "No, to the contrary, I thought that by getting accepted to such a prestigious school, I could solve my father's problems and become his pride. I hoped to realize the dream he never had been able to realize for himself, and I thought I would live up to becoming his favorite son."
T: "How do you feel about that now?"
C: "I feel cheated, nearly ashamed of myself . . . rejected, as if I had been a fool. I began to hate my father, but in a strange way I also felt superior to him."
T: "Can you describe more?"

C: "Maybe I felt that he was stupid and limited, and unable to appreciate my success. He probably began to feel inferior . . . or maybe envious . . . That is what my mother told me, that I did something he never even thought of allowing himself to do."

Mr. C's motivation to achieve was based on the wish to be able to compensate the father and regain a special relationship that was interrupted due to the father's illness. When he realized that he had failed to reach his father through his educational achievements, this very intelligent man maintained the narcissistic-masochistic fantasy that he was both a loser and a superior who could control and remain untouched by his father's cruelty and rejections. He remained angry, detached, and envious.

Case vignette

Mr. R, a man in his late forties who had began to suffer from episodes of such severe depression that his successful professional career was in jeopardy, took pride in being able to stay married to his extraordinarily humiliating, aggressive, impulsive, and unpredictably moody wife. He said that he deeply loved his wife, despite the fact that she both privately and publicly ridiculed, criticized, and counteracted him and periodically spent time away from him with different lovers. Secretly he nourished the idea that he was the only man who really understood, cared for, and was able to love this woman, and he was devoted to sacrificing himself to be able to succeed in what her father and two previous husbands had been unable to do, to give her love and understanding. To his therapist, Mr. R explained that his wife, due to her past marital experiences and growing up with a very inconsiderate father, just was unable to understand the effects of her actions. Several months later Mr. R revealed that no woman had previously made him feel so admired, important, strong, and attractive as his wife before they were married. By being supportive, understanding, and faithful toward his wife, Mr. R hoped that he would be able to regain such position and again experience the male strength, superiority, and attractiveness that his wife's admiration evoked in him.

Further into the therapy, Mr. R began to connect his feelings of depression with a growing awareness of his own experiences of constraints, guilt, and sacrifices in his marriage. He also became aware of his own rage toward his wife, which helped him to gain a more realistic understanding of her problems and his own role in the marriage. This also helped Mr. R to develop a protective distance to his wife's hurtful attacks and behavior, which actually turned out to have a calming influence on his wife's behavior. As he began to have more mutual and enjoyable moments with his wife, he decided to stay in the marriage.

Reactions to Criticism   Low capacity to discriminate NPD and high presence in other personality disorders prompted the decision to exclude reactions to criticism from the *DSM-IV* NPD criteria (Gunderson, Ronningstam, & Smith, 1991). However, recent research on self-esteem regulation (Baumeister et al., 1993; Morf & Rhodewalt, 2001; Rhodewalt et al., 1998; Smalley & Stake, 1996; see above) has helped to identify specific patterns that discriminate narcissistic reactivity. In general, ego threats disrupt self-regulatory effectiveness in people with high self-esteem. Narcissistic people tend to interpret tasks and events as opportunities to show off, to demonstrate their superiority, and to compete with others. When criticized, they tend to react in various ways: They ward off intolerable criticism or threats by overestimating their own contributions, by ignoring or devaluing the critique or the person who criticizes, or by aggressively counterarguing or defending themselves; they also use self-aggrandizing strategies and self-illusion to boost positive feedback, commit to unrealistic goals, and take exaggerated credit for a success. Studies that have focused specifically on aggressive and violent reactions (Baumeister et al., 1996; Bushman & Baumeister, 1998; Papps & O'Carroll, 1998; Rhodewalt & Morf, 1998) all support the observation that people with high narcissism tend to have strong aggressive and violent reactions to threats to their sense of superiority or self-esteem. Aggressive reactions to criticism may be more or less controlled and obvious—ranging from cognitive reconstructions of events and subtle, well-hidden feelings of disdain or contempt, to intense aggressive argumentativeness, criticism, and rage outbursts, to more or less controlled aggressive and violent behavior. Intense emotional reactions such as rage and shame reflect both shifting levels of self-esteem and affect dysregulation (Rhodewalt et al., 1998; see below). Such reactions also differentiate NPD from antisocial and hypomanic people who are less prone to reactions and affectively more stable (Morey & Jones 1998).

Summary—Self-esteem Dysregulation   The main overt characteristics of narcissistic peoples' self-esteem regulation center around grandiosity, which is expressed in an inner sense of superiority and uniqueness and in grandiose fantasies of being the best, and powerful, attractive, admired, and so forth. The more noticeable manifest behavioral signs of grandiosity are self-centered and self-referential behavior and a boastful or pretentious attitude. Admiring attention from others serves to protect and enhance the grandiose self-experience, and narcissistic people make various more or less oblivious or obvious efforts to gain such supportive attention. The most important sign of narcissistic self-esteem dysregulation and consequential to the grandiose self-experience are the various strong reactions to criticism, defeats, or other threats to self-esteem. As mentioned above, manifestations of such reactions can range from subtle internal reevaluations, to active self-aggrandizing and self-protecting behavior, to more or less intense feelings of rage and shame (see below). In summary, self-esteem dysregulation involves

- a sense of superiority and uniqueness (Ronningstam & Gunderson, 1990)
- exaggeration of talents and achievements (Rhodewalt & Morf, 1998; Ronningstam & Gunderson, 1990)
- grandiose fantasies (Ronningstam & Gunderson, 1990)
- self-centered and self-referential behavior (Ronningstam & Gunderson, 1990)
- boastful and pretentious attitude (Ronningstam & Gunderson, 1990)
- need for admiring attention (Ronningstam & Gunderson, 1990)
- strong reactions to criticism and defeat (Morey & Jones, 1998; Rhodewalt & Morf, 1998)

Affect Regulation

People with NPD are challenged both by the presence of strong affects, especially rage, shame, and envy, and by the low tolerance of the nature and intensity of such feelings. This is especially evident in their difficulties modulating affects and their proneness to self-criticism and sensitivity to experiencing failures in maintaining inner control. Excessive, uncontrollable rage outbursts or proneness to self-shaming and extreme reactions to both success and humiliation are signs of such affect dysregulation. In addition, as mentioned above, certain aspects of narcissistic people's affect regulation and reactivity also reflect shifts in self-esteem (Morey & Jones, 1998). Narcissistic people are hypersensitive and prone to rapidly interpreting situations as either narcissistically rewarding or as threatening or humiliating. However, there are notable differences in expressions of such hypersensitivity. While some people may appear stoic, cold, and unemotional, obsessionally preoccupied with details, or detached and avoidant, others come across as emotionally lively, reactive and intensive, and even erratic or dramatic. An inability to acknowledge and communicate feelings is a common sign of affect dysregulation, especially among intelligent and ambitious narcissistic people.

Modell (1975, 1980) considered noncommunication of affects to be the most outstanding characteristic for a certain group of narcissistic patients. Because affects represent seeking and needing others, this grandiose illusion of self-sufficiency and noncommunication serves as a defense, like a cocoon, motivated by fear of closeness and intrusion from others. By not communicating affects at all, the patient is obviously not relating, and he or she acts as if the therapist/analyst is not there. The patient may also relate in a more subtle and empty way with false affects to induce his or her own feelings in the therapist/analyst. According to Modell, this is a way to omnipotently control the feelings of others or to create an illusion of inner mastery. In other words, such affect noncommunication serves to regulate self-esteem and maintain inner control. The term alexithymia, that is, having no words for emotions, has been used to capture the inability to use affects for information processing (Krystal, 1998; McDougall, 1985; Nemiah & Sifneos, 1970). The person is unable to identify, name, differentiate, and feel his or her own feelings, either because of unawareness or because of inability to distinguish physical and affect states such as happiness, excitement, sadness, anxiety, and anger. The person may be able to identify feelings in others but not in himself or herself. The awareness of such deficit may be embedded in chronic feelings of shame and contribute to an underlying intangible or vague sense of inferiority.

Case vignette

A painful realization was made by a young woman whose boyfriend had just left her: "I see others attach to each other and fall in love

but I can't," she said. "I say to myself, 'They are stupid and silly, I
have more important things to do, I am superior because I don't
get involved in such things,' but deep inside I realize that they have
something I do not have, or that I can't do. I seem to be able to do
and achieve everything I can think of, but I don't know what love
and affection are. I just get angry or feel bored when I am dating
somebody or trying to become friends with someone. I make a lot
of effort, but the more I try, the more I feel envious and ashamed
that there is something I am not able to do."

Anger and Rage   Aggression and its variations—irritability, resentment,
anger, vindictiveness, rage, and hatred—have historically been one of the
most significant features in pathological narcissism. Striking expressions,
such as aggressive argumentativeness, criticism and outbursts, acts of
sadism, revenge, and destructiveness are usually associated with narcissistic disorders. As mentioned above, studies have verified the connection
between narcissism and emotional reactivity and the fact that narcissistic
people indeed have subtle as well as intense aggressive, hostile, and even
violent reactions to threats to their egos and self-esteem (Baumeister,
Smart, Boden,1996; Bushman & Baumeister, 1998; Papps, O'Carroll,
1998; Rhodewalt & Morf, 1998). While the view of aggression as a motivational proactive agent for assertiveness and mastery in the development
of normal narcissism has been less disputed (see chapter 2 this volume), a
major disagreement regarding aggression in pathological narcissism concerns whether it is an inherited constitutional drive (O. Kernberg, 1984,
1992) or a reaction to frustration, threats, and injury to the self (Kohut,
1972). This discord still has major diagnostic as well as treatment implications for pathological narcissism and NPD.

O. Kernberg (1984, 1992), on the one hand, described the psychopathology of aggression in the borderline personality organization in general
and in NPD with a pathological grandiose self-structure in particular. He
outlined a differential diagnostic system for vicissitudes and degrees of
severity of rage and hatred, and related aggression to degrees of self-inte-
gration and to levels of ego and superego pathology as well as to qualities
in object relations. As such, aggression as an affect has, according to O.
Kernberg, a motivational function and links self-object representations
into internalized object relations associated to primarily frustrating experiences. Self-esteem regulation is understood in a dynamic context to the

extent that more or less primitive aggression, expressed overtly toward others or internally vis-à-vis the self, is contributing to a sense of superiority. Masochism, sadism, malignant narcissism, controlled self-destructiveness, and suicidal behavior and systematic expressions of rage and violent behavior (see below) are variations of such aggression.

Kohut (1972), on the other hand, viewed human aggression in general as a constructive motivational force, but when attached to a grandiose self and an archaic omnipotent object aggression becomes dangerous and destructive. He described *narcissistic rage*, a specific form of rage that represents one of two reactions (the other being shamefaced withdrawal) in a narcissistically shame-prone or vulnerable individual in response to a narcissistic injury. This type of rage, which can range from deep chronic grudge to archaic violent fury, is related to the need for absolute control of the environment, "the need for revenge, for righting a wrong, for undoing a hurt by whatever means, and a deeply anchored, unrelenting compulsion in the pursuit of all these aims" (p. 380). It is based on a desire to turn a passive experience of victimization into an active act of inflicting injury onto others. Narcissistic rage is archaic in nature and characterized by relentlessness, sharp reasoning, lack of empathy, and unforgivingness. As such, it is strongly motivated by an effort to restore and maintain self-esteem. However, narcissistic rage can also involve self-protection (Dodes, 1990) and can serve to restore a sense of internal power and safety. As such, it is associated with self-preservation and entitlement and to the urge to destroy any interference to such rights (Murray, 1964). In more severely disturbed people the narcissistic rage might be associated with envy and an urge to attack the intolerable good qualities and desirable assets of others to maintain self esteem. Turned toward the self, this type of rage can lead to suicidal ideations and severe deadly self attacks.

The relationship between aggressive affects and actions is especially complex in narcissistic people. Seemingly aggressive acts, such as rejecting or destructive behavior, are not necessarily motivated or accompanied by aggressive affects, and aggressive feelings are not necessarily accompanied by aggressive actions. Rizzuto and colleagues (Rizzuto, Meissner, & Buie, 2004) differentiated between an aggressive action that serves to overcome external or internal obstacles and an aggressive affect that has its source or motivation in personal historical, internal, or external context. They suggested that "motivations for angry and rageful feelings have their own dynamic sources that may be independent of the aggressive intrapsychic or external activity" (p. 117). For example, aggressive affective reactions to narcissistic injury or threats to the self-esteem, such as narcissistic rage, serve to protect or enhance the self-esteem and to ward off such danger and may not have an aggressive aim per se. A narcissistic person in treatment may deny feeling angry or behaving aggressively or may react by feeling surprised, hurt, or humiliated, or paradoxically even angry in response to inquires of whether he might feel angry. This makes it especially important to understand such motivational as well as affect and self-esteem regulatory contexts when helping the narcissistic individuals in identifying their own motivation and aim behind functional, behavioral, and emotional expressions of aggression. In addition, feelings related to aggression may be intertwined with or overshadowed by other feelings such as shame, self-scorn, inferiority, and so on, which call for a complex and intricate exploration and differentiation.

Case vignette

A young man spoke emphatically with the assigned therapist after having attempted to commit suicide:

P: "Just so you know this: I don't 'do feelings,' so don't make any efforts to talk to me about any emotional crap!"
T: "Maybe you have reasons not to feel feelings?"
P: "Give me one single reason why I should feel feelings. They interfere with my studies and hobbies, disrupt my sleep, and ruin my relationships. That's why I don't do feelings!!"
T: "Right now you sound angry, and you have just made a suicide attempt . . . "
P: "Yeah . . . so what . . . ?!"
T: "Do you think that your anger could have something to do with your suicide attempt?"
P: "Absolutely not!! It was an entirely logical and intellectual decision, the only problem was that I underestimated the necessary and optimal dosage for killing myself."
T: "So maybe that makes you angry."
P: "Yes, it certainly does!!"

This ambitious young man, who had been facing an intolerable realization that he was unable to live up to his own exceptionally high academic standards, found it too demeaning to admit having angry feelings. Not feeling feelings at all was an important aspect of his sense of superiority and inner control. He also denied that feelings of anger were involved in the self-destructive act of attempting suicide. Such denial probably helped this man to avoid feeling the despair, worthlessness, and self-directed rage that might have preceded his suicide attempt.

Shame   Feelings of shame have been specifically associated with narcissism (Morrison, 1989). Shame is evoked by "a sense of contempt or disgust by the Other and the experience of some defect in the self" (Pulver 1999, p. 393) (see chapter 2 this volume). It is not the shame itself but rather an early developing inefficient capacity to autoregulate or interactively regulate this potent affect that is psychopathogenic (Schore, 1998). Shame is a response to an environmental feedback suggesting incompetence, inefficacy, and the inability to influence, predict, or comprehend an event that the child expected to be able to control or understand (Broucek, 1982). As such, feelings of shame are closely related to self-evaluation and self-esteem regulation. Tangney (1990, 1991, 1995) has in her extensive studies on shame identified several significant characteristics: Shame is a debilitating emotion that often serves to paralyze the self. It can be overwhelming and devastatingly painful and involve the entire self, leading, at least temporarily, to a crippling of adaptive self-functions. Shame involves a significant shift in self-perception, accompanied by a sense of exposure, a sense of shrinking, and feelings of worthlessness and powerlessness. In other words, the perception of one's own feelings of shame tends to lower an individual's self-esteem. Shame proneness is also related to a number of problematic behaviors such as procrastination (Fee & Tangney, 2000), suicidal behavior (Hastings et al., 2001), depression (Tangney, Wagner & Gramzow,1992), and narcissism and pathological narcissistic defenses (Gramzow & Tangney, 1992).

Because shame is an acutely painful affective experience, the pain of shame in itself may also motivate anger, hostility, or humiliated fury (H. B. Lewis, 1971; Tangney, Wagner, Fletcher, and Gramzow, 1992; Tangney, Wagner, Hill-Barlow, Marshcall, & Gramzow, 1996). Such anger can be directed toward the self, but because shame typically involves the imagery of a real or imagined rejecting, disapproving other, shame-based anger can easily be directed in retaliation toward others and serve defensive functions. By redirecting anger, the person regains a sense of control and mastery that is impaired by shameful experiences (H. B. Lewis, 1971) and gets relief from the global self-condemning and debilitating experience of shame. Several studies have shown that shame proneness is consistently correlated with anger arousal, suspiciousness, resentment, irritability, a tendency to blame others for negative events, and indirect expression of hostility (Tangney & Fischer, 1995).

Shame has been strongly associated with the urge to hide and the impact of shame in interpersonal relationships has usually been overlooked. Nevertheless, the tendencies to express humiliated fury triggered by shame and to externalize blame usually cause severe difficulties in interpersonal relationships. It can lead to irrational and aggressive shame–blame cycles with subsequent rejections from the targeted or blamed person (H. B. Lewis, 1971). Because the distress and pain associated to shame tend to shift the person's attention inward, shame feelings also tend to have a negative impairing effect on the capacity for empathy and for concern and connection with other people (Tangney, 1995, pp. 129–130).

Feelings of shame can remain hidden and be effectively rationalized or defended against. Consequently, shame has usually been associated with the shy, covert, and vulnerable narcissistic personality (see below). In addition, the significance of the shame-inducing/triggering experiences may be bypassed, denied, or even totally unknown (Tangney, 1991). In other words, the presence and impact of shame can easily be overlooked in the evaluation and treatment of people with narcissistic disorders. However, the connection between shame and anger, hostility and blaming makes the presence of shame more manifest and a central feeling also in the arrogant narcissistic personality.

Envy The connection between narcissism and envy has been especially difficult to clarify because awareness of one's own feelings of envy, in and by itself, tends to lower self-esteem and evoke feelings of shame. In other words, a strong internal readiness to deny feelings of envy, usually accompanied by social reinforcements of such denial, makes envy a vexatious inquiry. In psychoanalytic studies, envy was considered rooted in constitutional aggression. According to M. Klein (1957), early primitive envy represents a malignant and severe form of innate aggression. Rosenfeld (1987) suggested that the narcissistic character structure is a defense against envy and dependency. Envy-prone people who experience goodness in another person feel the goodness to be painfully insufficient and resent both their own dependency upon the other and the other's control over the goodness. Envy is defined as hatred directed toward good objects. Compared to "regular" hatred, in which the good object is protected and

the bad object is attacked, in hatred with primitive envy another's goodness is experienced as a threat to the person's own grandiosity or idealized self-experience, and the goodness is destroyed. In other words, by
attacking the good object, the person is trying to ward off feelings of pain,
vulnerability, dependency, and defectiveness that are evoked by recognizing the threatening goodness in another person. Envy can destroy the
possibility for hope and diminish capacity for enjoyment.

Barth (1988) suggested a relationship between narcissistic injury and
envious feelings, such that envy can be both a stimulus for and a result
of self-esteem dysregulation. In other areas, envy may represent both an
attempt to avoid painful injury to one's self-esteem and an effort to maintain a positive self-esteem. In a cycle of self-esteem dysregulation, feelings of inadequacy and/or inferiority and envious rage—which includes
a wish to destroy either the possessor or that which is possessed—are
followed by self-criticism and shame for such hateful, hostile, and greedy
feelings. In this process, "the ability to value oneself and one's possession
(including personal characteristics, feelings of being loved, personal and
professional achievement, etc.) is often destroyed." (p. 201). Hence, "envy
not only makes it difficult for the individual to appreciate (take in) what
the envied person offers, but it also interferes with the individual's ability
to appreciate what he or she already has" (p. 201). Rage and greed that
accompany envy can represent attempts to restore or protect self-esteem.
"The rage may be empowering, may help to compensate for feelings of
inadequacy which trigger the envy in the first place" (p. 202). However,
Barth also noted that feelings of rage paradoxically also may increase the
feelings of shame.

Envy is always disguised, hardly ever appearing in a straightforward
manner (Etchegoyen, Benito, & Rabih, 1987). The expressions of envy
in social and interpersonal contexts can be extremely subtle and undermining, ranging from discrete spoiling behavior and withholding what
a person needs, such as praise, empathy, warmth, attention, admiration, support, or comfort, to actively spoiling or destroying the object
(Schwartz-Salant, 1982). While envy usually is associated with material
possessions, social status, personal attributes, and professional status and
accomplishments, paradoxically envy can also apply to another person's
capacity to tolerate *not* having something or managing frustration related
to absence and lacking. Powerful envy can be expressed in feelings of
continually being wronged or mistreated by the object (Moser-Ha,
2001). Malicious envy, which is followed by pain and feelings of infe-

riority, involves a wish to eliminate or destroy what one is not able to possess (Habimana & Masse 2000), and destructive efforts can even be directed toward the other person's happiness, future accomplishments, and relationships.

While narcissistic people readily deny feelings of envy toward others, they often report intense reactions to the perception of others' envy (Ronningstam & Gunderson, 1990). In other words, the belief that other people envy them because of their special talents or unique qualities is associated with suspicious and hostile reactions. Such reactions may remain hidden or be overtly expressed, depending upon the nature and level of the individual's narcissistic functioning. On the one hand, while the preoccupation with others' envy may represent a projection of one's own intolerable envy onto other people, it may also be a sign of hypersensitivity and a perception of other people's envy as a threat to one's own self-esteem and grandiose self-experience, that is, a belief that others are going to criticize or destroy what one can do or have. On the other hand, the sensitivity to others' envy can also be associated with a particular superior awareness of others' attention, self-righteous anger, and even a hidden sadistic satisfaction in causing a sense of inferiority and painful feelings in others.

Mood and Hypochondria   Affect dysregulation with sharp mood variations and rapid shifts is closely related to and sometimes misinterpreted as mood disorders. However, in narcissistic people, such mood swings, that is, irritability, cynicism or brief reactive depression, or excitement, optimism, and confidence, reflect shifting levels of self-esteem and are highly dependent on external support for self-esteem or on perceived threats to the grandiose self. Sharp mood variations in response to such threats can also include states of hypomania or sudden explosive rage (Cooper, 1998).

Psychosomatic reactions or disorder, periodic substance abuse, hypochondria, and preoccupation with the body can in some narcissistic people represent a regression in or replacement of regular affects (Krystal, 1998), especially in the context of threats and challenges to the self-esteem. For other people with less severe narcissistic disorder, the inability to feel feelings may represent a defense, that is, a sense of superior perfection and control over especially strong feelings that are considered inappropriate. This, in turn, may be attached to feelings of vulnerability, lack of control, and imperfection. In addition, the presence of strong feelings of shame or shame-based guilt may impair the capacity to identify and feel feelings.

Summary—Affect Dysregulation   The most significant characteristic of narcissistic affect dysregulation is the predominance of feelings of anger, shame, and envy and the individual's strong proneness to react intensively with such feelings to perceived humiliations and threats to self-esteem. While anger reactions, ranging from silent contempt to overt hostility and explosive rage outbursts, are often but not always noticeable and obvious, the feelings of shame and envy are usually more hidden or indirectly expressed, such as in the tendency to blame or in reactions to the perception of others' envy. Mood variations, including depression, irritability, elation, or hypomania, reflect shifting levels of self-esteem. In summary, affect dysregulation involves

- strong feelings of shame and envy (Cooper, 1998; Cooper & Ronningstam, 1992; O. Kernberg, 1998b)
- intense aggressive reactions to threats to self-esteem (Morey & Jones, 1998; Rhodewalt & Morf, 1998)
- sharp mood variations (Cooper, 1998; Cooper & Ronningstam, 1992)
- intense reactions to the perception of others' envy (Ronningstam & Gunderson, 1990)

Interpersonal Relationships

Interpersonal relations represent the most consequential area of functioning for people with narcissistic disorders. Not only are they sensitive to and reliant upon support and feedback from others for their self-knowledge and self-esteem regulation, but also they actively seek admiring attention from others and use the social environment and other people to enhance their self-esteem (Rhodewalt et al., 1998; Ronningstam & Gunderson, 1990). On the other hand, other people also represent a constant threat to the narcissistic individual's self-experience and inasmuch as others can make narcissistic individuals feel superior, entitled, and confident, they can also contribute to their feeling extremely ashamed, inferior, worthless, irritable, and enraged.

Problems with commitment and difficulties in taking on others' perspective, interpreting others, and understanding and tolerating others' feelings, combined with entitlement and unrealistic expectations of others, often lead to severe interpersonal failures and conflicts and to potential isolation. In other words, the interpersonal arena tends to become a major battlefield for narcissistic individuals. Such problems are also the most serious obstacle to engaging in and benefiting from treatment.

Entitlement Officially defined as unreasonable expectations of especially favorable treatment or automatic compliance with one's expectations (*DSM-IV*), entitlement may either stem from a sense of grandiose self-righteousness or function as a defense against feelings of envy, guilt, shame, depression, and threat of closeness (Moses & Moses-Hrushovski, 1990). A sense of entitlement was the most reliable and valid indicator of narcissism in a study by Dowson (1992). Expressions of entitlement can range from infuriated reactions—irritability, hostile rejecting, or vindictive behavior—to feeling surprised, hurt, unappreciated, unfairly treated, or even exploited. Entitlement is closely related to a passive attitude and lack of self-initiative (Kerr, 1985) and to an experience of not getting as much as one deserves (Havens, 1993). It can also be associated with expectations or hopes for reparation of past damages or correction of injustices (Moses & Moses-Hrushovski, 1990). An expectation that things should come easily and be provided by others often comes with negative or even shameful feelings toward the requirement of one's own efforts. Further explorations of people's feelings of entitlement may reveal a striking contrast between inner experiences of defectiveness, undesirability, or worthlessness and an overt special entitled attitude of unrealistic rights, expectations, and exemptions (Cohen, 1988). Entitlement in such a dynamic context may have its roots in unmodulated aggression and harsh judgmental self-criticism.

Case vignette

Mr. N, a professional in his mid forties, felt that it was his employer's task to provide him with meaningful and interesting work. When talking with one of his successful friends, who owned his own business, he expressed deep dissatisfaction with his present employer. The friend advised him to either get further education, develop an area of own expertise, or open his own consulting business. Mr. N got very upset and stopped all further communications with his friend. Several months later Mr. N revealed to his therapist his fear of failure and deep feelings of insecurity when facing new tasks, especially if they required training and acquiring new skills. He also admitted feeling envious, intimidated, and afraid in interactions with more assertive and successful colleagues. By having his employer outline his work tasks, Mr. N felt attended to and specially treated. It was as if this sense of attention and specialness made him feel more competent at the same time as it protected him from his own underlying envy and insecurity.

Paradoxically, and despite strong feelings of entitlement, narcissistic people may also feel ambivalent and suffer from an inability to feel that they fully deserve what seems to be the basic rights and conditions in the lives of other people. This type of "nonentitlement" (Kriegman, 1983) or compromised sense of fully deserving or doubts about deserving certain or even basic things in life is important to identify because it may underlie other exaggerated and unrealistic entitled strivings and attitudes that are more readily presented in the narcissistic individual.

A sense of exaggerated entitlement can also exist under a seemingly timid, compliant, or masochistic surface in people who present a willingness to attend to others while secretly feeling used, unrecognized, and resentful. Relevant for the treatment alliance is some narcissistic patients' expectation that the therapist should be able to "read their minds" and know and understand without having to verbalize what they think, feel, and want. Silence and withdrawal may be a reaction and expression of hurt omnipotence and passive aggression when such expectations are not met. Facing unfulfilled expectations can also evoke intense feelings of shame.

Empathy   Lack of empathy has been considered one of the main characteristics of narcissistic people, along with grandiosity. Because they often come across as ignorant of and even unsympathetic to other people's feelings, it has readily been assumed that they also lack empathy. This general notion, also held by *DSM-IV*, seems to ignore that both cognitive and emotional as well as interpersonal functions influence the pattern of and capacity for empathic processing. However, so far no studies have focused specifically on the relationship of self-esteem, affect dysregulation, and narcissistic interpersonal functioning to empathic processing.

Fonagy, Gergely, Jurist, and Target (2002) identified neuropsychological origins of limited empathic processing located in the amygdala and orbitofrontal cortex. Of relevance for narcissistic empathic dysfunctioning is the impaired capacity for understanding one's own emotions and reactions. In addition, impairment or disconnection in interpersonal interpretive functioning also contributes to low empathy. "The individual might experience affect in relation to another's distress but this is inappropriately or inadequately linked to a representation of the belief and intentional state of that person" (p. 139). This corresponds to the narcissistic individual's tendencies to misinterpret states and emotions in others and to a disconnection between cognitive and emotional interpretative processes.

Several narcissistic features interfere with empathy. Low affect tolerance is incompatible with empathic processing (Schore, 1994). The perception of others' states may evoke both intolerable feelings in the narcissistic person and a sense of incompetence and helplessness that seriously interferes with the capacity for empathy. Proneness to shame tends to impair the capacity for other-oriented empathic concern (Tangney, 1995), and feelings of both shame and envy are accompanied by the urge to withdraw, which hinders active interpersonal processing of empathy. Biased self-perception, egocentricity, and self-preoccupation interfere with the ability for perspective taking and emotional resonance. By nature, entitlement and the readiness for self-serving expectations in others are incompatible with empathy. In addition, self-enhancement and other strategies to protect and increase self-esteem are also incompatible with interpersonal orientation and empathy (Campbell, Reeder, Sedikides, & Elliot, 2000).

Case vignette

A man in his mid-twenties experienced extraordinary difficulties in interactions with other people. Despite being very intelligent, well-behaved, and intellectually aware of social rules, he repeatedly encountered situations with others that he found extremely confusing. He described one such situation: "I run into this woman; she was very attractive and she started to talk to me in a nice, soft, and somewhat seductive voice which I found totally out of place given the context—we were at gasoline station. I began to feel confused, she obviously was interested in me, maybe she was trying to 'pick me up.' I found her very attractive and appealing but I got afraid because I did not know what to say to her and I was not sure about what she really wanted or even what I wanted myself. I felt too guilty to just walk away; she obviously wanted something from me. I had to pay for my gasoline, and when I did not respond to her she looked at me as if I had hurt her, which made me feel even more guilty and uncomfortable. I just wanted to pay and get out of the situation as soon as possible."

This young man presented several of the main features of severely impaired empathy; that is, difficulties feeling and understanding others' intentions and emotional states, difficulties reading others' facial expressions, difficulties reading, understanding and regulating his own body state and affects such as sexual and emotional excitement, fear, shame, and insecurity, and difficulties taking on the perspective and feelings of another person while maintaining awareness and control of his own affects and experiences. Consequently, interpersonal interactions tend to become very taxing on his self-esteem and he often encountered feeling confused, cheated, betrayed, criticized, or rejected. This young man usually preferred either to dominate and take charge of interactions with others and pursue his own interests and intentions or to avoid other people totally. Nevertheless, despite these problems, he also demonstrated a capacity to notice and to some degree evaluate his difficulties and to feel guilt for his problems in understanding and responding to others.

The clinical presentation of impaired empathic capacity in narcissistic people may range from tuned-in unassuming interest, to misunderstanding and confusion, to subtle inattention or inability to listen, to complete oblivious insensitivity, to superior intellectual demonstrations of capability to identify mental states and feelings in others. In addition, empathic dysfunctions may be expressed either as efforts to control others' inner states or as overtly disdainful, critical, or aggressive reactions toward others' feelings and distress, or, in more severe forms of pathological narcissism, as attempts to con, manipulate, or emotionally exploit others based on identification of those others' inner state and distress. In diagnostic evaluation and treatment planning with narcissistic people, it is of crucial importance to differentiate between emotional, interpersonal, and cognitive origins of empathic dysfunctioning, as well as to identify the specific developmental origin and the pattern of attachment and attunement that could have contributed to the specific empathic impairment.

Case vignette

One young woman said, "I see my friend crying over the most stupid thing, something that does not really concern her. For instance, she cried because her friend's mother had died. I got angry with her—there was no reason for her to cry because of that. Sometimes she may cry for more valid reasons, like when her dog died. I can understand that, but I still cannot tolerate it. I get angry and resentful. I never behave like this myself."

Further exploration in psychotherapy revealed that this woman actually felt envious of her friend who was able to cry so easily. Her own father had died when she was 9, and she had never been able to either cry or fully grieve. Instead, she had adopted a stoic attitude, convincing herself and others that the loss of her father really did not bother her. Her friend's reactions evoked her own sense of loss, which made her feel weak and vulnerable, ashamed of herself and, as a result, resentful toward her friend. In addition, her anger also accompanied a sense of temporary superiority vis-à-vis her friend.

Some narcissistic people present as extremely sensitive with seemingly good or even superior ability to identify feelings and intentions in others. However, these people often lack the ability to respond and relate to people who seek their genuine attention or empathy.

Case vignette

A wife described her husband: "When we got married I believed my husband was one of the most empathic men I ever met. He helped me understand and outgrow my problematic relationships to my sister and brothers by pointing out how their behavior made me react. He was particularly helpful to me in explaining the motivation behind my mother's irrational behavior and extreme reactions, which always have been very embarrassing and puzzling to all of us. It was the same with our friends; he could quickly identify people's experience, motives, and feelings and he was amazingly accurate.

But gradually I noticed that he was detached and seemingly indifferent to distress in our relationship or to the specific difficulties I
experienced. To my surprise, I found him totally unable to see or
experience my perspective. It was as if he was a different person.
When I told him about my feelings or sought his support, he got
numb and seemed to tune out. Sometimes he got irritated and even
angry. I felt shocked and confused by his insensitivity."

Arrogance, control, and hostility   Some narcissistic people present themselves as strikingly arrogant and haughty (Ronningstam & Gunderson,
1990); others might initially appear more timid but gradually present
more hidden and specific areas of disdainful or pejorative attitudes.
Morey and Jones (1998) identified expressions of both active and passive
interpersonal hostility. The degree and type of hostility can vary from less
obvious passive-aggressive behavior to overtly belittling, exploitative, or
sadistic behavior, especially toward subordinates. They also mentioned
the need for interpersonal control as an important aspect of the narcissistic individual's relational pattern, that is, an unempathic, detached
involvement with self-serving purposes. The motive for such strivings can
stem both from a sense of superiority vis-à-vis others and from a need
to protect self-esteem and self-cohesiveness from threatening or unexpected disorganizing experiences. In addition, interpersonal dominance
is used as a strategy to manage hostility and regulate self-esteem (Raskin
et al., 1991). Bach (1977b) noticed that language and words can be used
for narcissistic strivings in interpersonal relationships less for the purpose
of communicating and understanding and more for a manipulative function "to frighten or to soothe, to distance or to merge, to control or to be
controlled " (p. 219).

Interpersonal Commitment   The inability to engage in long-term commitments has primarily been associated with the lack of tolerance for the
challenge to self-esteem and the intensity of affects involved in a deep
long-term mutual relationship. Cooper (1998) noted an interpersonal
relational pattern of early enthusiasm that is followed by disappointment.
Lack of commitment is an indicator of more long-term, enduring forms
of NPD (Ronningstam et al., 1995) and associated with poor prognoses
and absence of change. Lack of commitment can also be an expression
of a more severe narcissistic disturbance in the context of irresponsible,

actively exploitative, or even corruptive interpersonal behavior. On the other hand, a capacity for long-term commitment to others, even in the presence of other severe signs of narcissistic pathology, points toward changeability and better prognosis, because it enables the person to commit to family, to work, or to a treatment team.

Exploitativeness   Exploitativeness, a feature associated with pathological narcissism and NPD and traditionally focused on privileges, material, or monetary gain, or personal or professional resources of others, did not distinguish narcissistic people in our studies (Ronningstam & Gunderson, 1990, 1991; Gunderson & Ronningstam, 2001). Exploitative behavior also did not differentiate NPD from BPD or ASPD in the study by Holdwick, Hilsenroth, Castlebury, and Blais (1998). It seems important to differentiate among (a) the more obvious, active, and consciously exploitative behavior found in antisocial and psychopathic individuals, (b) the need-fulfilling exploitative behavior found in borderline patients, and (c) the more passive, manipulative, and entitled, emotionally focused exploitative behavior that serves to support or enhance self-esteem in narcissistic individuals. It also seems important to differentiate exploitative behavior resulting from aggressive entitlement, that is, the sense of the right to pick on, blame, and misuse others, and that resulting from revengeful or malignant entitlement (O. Kernberg, 1984), that is, the right to retaliate, parasitize, or violate others. The dynamics behind such entitlement differ from that leading to exploitative behavior.

Summary—Interpersonal Relationships   Narcissistic individuals are usually identified by their specific interpersonal pattern with a more or less overtly arrogant and haughty attitude, and entitled and controlling behavior. Hostility can range from subtle passive-aggressive behavior to sadistic or explosive behavior. Inability to commit to others is the sign of a long-term, enduring NPD. Specific attention should be paid to the range of empathic dysfunctions and varieties in expressions of impaired empathic processing that can be found in narcissistic individuals. In summary, narcissistic interpersonal relationships involve

- arrogant and haughty behavior (Ronningstam & Gunderson, 1990)
- entitlement (Cooper, 1998; Dowson, 1992; Ronningstam & Gunderson, 1990;)

- impaired empathic capacity (Cooper, 1998)
- interpersonal control and hostility (Morey & Jones, 1998)
- lack of sustained commitment to others (Cooper, 1998; Ronningstam et al. 1995)

Narcissistic Personality Disorder—The Shy Type

The "shy narcissist" is now a common label for people with a different clinical presentation of NPD, and several reports have outlined the features and diagnostic criteria for this type of NPD (Akhtar, 1997, 2003; Cooper, 1998; Cooper & Ronningstam, 1992; Dowson, 1992; Gabbard, 1989; Masterson, 1993). Although these specific expressions of narcissistic disorder are not yet included in the official *DSM-IV* criteria set, they are acknowledged as associated features. They include vulnerable self-esteem, feelings of shame, sensitivity and intense reactions of humiliation, hollowness, emptiness or disdain in response to criticism or defeat, and vocational irregularities due to difficulties tolerating criticism or competition (*DSM-IV*, p. 659; *DSM-IV-TR*, pp. 715–716). The identification of this group of NPD, also called the covert, hypervigilant, or "closet narcissist," stems from the recognition of the fragile, vulnerable self-structure in some narcissistic people and the role of shame in the development of pathological narcissism (Broucek, 1982). As mentioned above, this type of narcissistic patient appears quite different compared to those captured in the regular *DSM* criteria set: hypersensitive and self-effacing (Gabbard, 1989), inhibited and unassuming (Cooper & Ronningstam, 1992), and modest, humble, and seemingly uninterested in social success (Akhtar, 1997).

While clinical descriptions formed the foundation of this type, three studies confirm the presence of two facets in pathological narcissism. Wink (1991) found that narcissism divided into two factors, one implying grandiosity-exhibitionism and another vulnerability-sensitivity. Both were associated with conceit, self-indulgence, and disregard for others, but the vulnerability factor also captured anxiety and pessimism, introversion, defensiveness, anxiety, and vulnerability to life trauma. In another study, Hibbard (1992) correlated measures tapping both aggressive and vulnerable styles of narcissism, and shame, masochism, object relation, and social desirability. Results showed that narcissism consists of two different styles, a "phallic" grandiose style and a narcissistic vulnerable style.

Shame contributed to the major differences between these styles, correlating negatively with the grandiose style and positively with the more vulnerable style. Hibbard found that masochism has a narcissistic function because it correlates with shame-accompanied narcissism. J. D. C. Perry and Perry (2004) also gained support for the expression of narcissism on a fantasy level in their study of psychodynamic conflicts in NPD. They suggested that the use of autistic fantasy accompanying omnipotence and devaluation may also compensate for real action and accomplishment when a sense of failure, disappointment, or powerlessness is prominent.

Self-esteem Regulation

Avoiding ambitions and exposure to competitive and challenging situations is an important part of the shy narcissist's dysregulated self-esteem (Gabbard, 1989). This is in sharp contrast to the arrogant narcissist, who seeks out opportunities for self-exposure and competition and often comes across as self-assured, knowledgeable, and competent. Shy narcissistic personalities usually hide their grandiosity. Grandiose desires are not expressed and acted upon, and narcissistic pursuits are often performed on a fantasy level (Cooper & Ronningstam, 1992; Akhtar, 1997). In fact, their grandiose fantasies may be excessively compensatory, replacing actual achievements and interactions and compensating for inhibitions and the inability to expose and realize inner wishes and motivations. Gabbard (1989) suggested that "[a]t the core of their inner world is a deep sense of shame related to their secret wish to exhibit themselves in a grandiose manner" (p. 529). Both such feelings of excessive shame and the presence of a strict conscience (Akhtar, 1997) and harsh self-criticism tend to seriously inhibit shy narcissistic individuals, impair executive functioning, and force them to hide both grandiose strivings and actual ambitions, competence, and achievements.

Many people with the shy type of narcissistic disorder can actually be aware of the discrepancies between their grandiose view of themselves and wishes for their future, and their actual capacity and functioning. Such awareness may cause intense self-criticism, deep feelings of inferiority and shame, fear of failure in living up to grandiose aspirations, and an inability to appreciate their own actual achievements. Masterson (1993) noted that "closet narcissists" tend to idealize and invest in an omnipotent other person that come to represent their own grandiose self, while they themselves present a rather deflated and inadequate self.

It is a specific diagnostic challenge to differentiate among unrealistic grandiosity and grandiose fantasies, hidden ambitions, realistic capabilities and pursuits, and inhibitions due to shame or excessive self-criticism in these types of narcissistic patients. This often requires thorough explorations of people's self-experiences, which can reveal more complex or even paradoxical experiences of being special or exceptional. For instance, a person may take pride in being special in relation to his or her parents while at the same time feeling inferior, insecure, and resentful. Such hidden grandiosity and unconscious patterns of narcissistic self-esteem regulation may take a long time to explore and clarify in psychotherapy.

Case vignette

Ms. F, a timid, shy, and inhibited unmarried woman in her mid thirties, had decided, after several years in psychotherapy, to apply to law school and pursue a career as a lawyer. Since she was a teenager she had secretly nourished the dream of becoming a successful lawyer, like her father. When notified that she had been accepted, she had an unexpected and strong negative reaction: "This was not supposed to happen," she said. "I am not supposed to have a better life than my parents. I was raised to be neither seen nor heard. It was other people's privilege to have knowledge, to ask questions, to be part of an active life and pursue a meaningful career. My father told me that women would never make good lawyers and I believed him. I am breaking all the family rules by doing this. I feel like a fool."

Further explorations revealed that by pursuing her educational goals, Ms. F had exhibited a secret ambition that she felt was both inappropriate, forbidden, and shameful. However, she had also lost her position as the special and perfect, loyal, obedient, quiet, and supportive daughter who adhered to the unspoken family rules and attended to her parents' needs. This special position vis-à-vis her parents had contributed to a strong sense of pride and superiority, especially in relation to her more assertive and extravagant siblings, whom she secretly despised for their outlandish lifestyles. However, her position had also contributed to constrictions and inhibitions in her life. And now, when she had an agenda of her own, she suddenly felt insecure and self-critical, envious of her outgoing and successful siblings and enraged at her parents.

Affect Regulation

The shy narcissist is highly sensitive, has easily hurt feelings, and is prone to feeling ashamed, embarrassed, and humiliated, especially when confronted with the recognitions of unsatisfied needs or deficiencies in his or her capacities (Gabbard, 1989; Cooper, 1998). The exceptional sensitivity to exposure and attention, and accompanying overwhelming feelings of shame and anxiety, is one of the more specific features of this narcissistic type (Akhtar, 1997; Gabbard, 1989). Hypochondria, a sign of affect regression and expression of affects as somatic symptoms, serves defensive purposes to cover grandiosity, omnipotence, and masochism (Cooper, 1998; Akhtar, 1997). Unhappiness, pessimism, and a sense of lack of fulfillment, inner yearning, and waiting and hoping for recognition and changes to come are major characteristics of the inner affect state of this narcissist type (Akhtar, 1997; Hunt, 1995; Wink, 1991).

Interpersonal Relativeness

Shy narcissists are extremely attentive to others. They are hypersensitive and tend to pay specific attention to others' reactions to them, especially slights and criticism (Gabbard, 1989). Their capacity for empathy is compromised due to their envy, self-denigration, and extreme self-preoccupation. Shy narcissistic people often come across as empathic and sensitive, and they can appear interested in and even "tuned in" to other people. Some may even be capable of identifying feelings and inner experiences in others, that is, capable of empathic registration. Their unassuming shyness and wish to be noticed may mistakenly be perceived as a genuine interest in and capacity to care for others. However, they are equally unable to genuinely respond to others' needs and to involve themselves in enduring mutual personal relationships as their arrogant counterpart (Cooper & Ronningstam, 1992). Nevertheless, and contrary to the arrogant type, shy narcissistic individuals are able to feel remorse for their incapacity to empathize with others (Akhtar, 1997) and guilt caused by awareness of their shallowness and lack of concern for others (Cooper & Ronningstam, 1992). Akhtar (1997) also noticed that the shy narcissist has a stricter conscience and holds high moral standards with fewer tendencies for inconsistency and compromises of ethical values and rules. They may also be ambivalent toward their sense of entitlement, struggling with feelings of not deserving what they actually are entitled to, or

they may suppress exaggerated entitlement together with self-righteousness, aggression, and grandiosity behind a façade of shyness and aloofness
(Moses & Moses-Hrushovski, 1990).

Summary—The Shy Narcissistic Personality Disorder

From a diagnostic perspective, this subtype reflects characteristics of the
narcissistic, avoidant, and masochistic personality disorders. Because their
presentation is not easily recognizable, correct diagnosis usually requires
several sessions, or a period of psychotherapy. Self-esteem regulation
in shy narcissistic people is much more influenced by shaming, which
inhibits not only the expressions of grandiosity but also the individual's
pursuits of actual capabilities and opportunities in their lives. In other
words, unlike arrogant type, who is more openly aggressive, vocationally
involved, and actively seeking narcissistic gratification and self-enhancement, the shy narcissist is constricted both interpersonally and vocationally. The hypersensitivity and attentive readiness for slights and criticism
from others indicates an extreme vulnerability. In addition, the intense
feelings of shame increase interpersonal detachment and hiding, which
contribute to experiences of feelings of incompetence and isolation.
Although shy narcissists, because of their timid, kind, helpful and unassuming presentation, may be less involved in aggressive conflicts with
others, their shallowness, envy, and inability to genuinely and consistently
care for others cause other types of interpersonal conflicts and rejections.
In summary, shy NPD shares the following features with the arrogant
narcissistic type:

- sense of superiority and uniqueness
- lack of sustained commitment to others
- impaired capacity for empathy
- strong feelings of envy

Features exclusive for the shy narcissistic type include

- compensatory grandiose fantasies (Cooper & Ronningstam,
  1992)
- shame for ambitions and grandiosity (Gabbard, 1989; Akhtar,
  1997, 2003; Cooper & Ronningstam, 1992)
- shunning being the center of attention (Gabbard, 1989)

- hypersensitivity to slights, humiliation, and criticism (Gabbard, 1989)
- harsh self-criticism (Cooper & Ronningstam, 1992)
- proneness to intense shame reactions (Gabbard, 1989; Cooper & Ronningstam, 1992)
- interpersonal and vocational inhibitions (Gabbard, 1989; Cooper & Ronningstam, 1992)
- modesty, humility, and unassumingness (Akhtar, 1997, 2003)
- hypochondria (Akhtar, 1997, 2003; Cooper & Ronningstam, 1992)
- dysphoric affect state with unhappiness, pessimism, lack of fulfillment, yearning, and waiting (Akhtar, 1997, 2003; Wink, 1991)

Narcissistic Personality Disorder—The Psychopathic Type

Superego Regulation

An additional dimension of diagnostic importance for evaluating narcissistic disorders and NPD relates to moral and ethical values and functioning. Narcissistic individuals can be found among those who openly take pride in their high moral standards and who criticize and devalue people with different and "lower" sets of rules and values. In more extreme cases, the narcissistic person may even show intolerance and condemnation of others to highlight the virtue of his or her own superior ethics. Nevertheless, inconsistent and contradictory moral standards are most common. Narcissistic persons may have strict demands for ethical or professional perfectionism, especially in others, at the same time as they are ready to cut corners, be dishonest, compromise rules and standards, or even commit a crime, all in the service of protection of their self-image. Another less striking ethical compromise and a way to avoid feelings of shame and inferiority is the tendency to shift meanings and misrepresent or reconstruct events. Horowitz (1975) described this use of sliding meanings as "externalization of bad attributes and internalization of good attributes in order to stabilize self-concept. These operations serve distortion of reality and imply either a willingness to corrupt fidelity to reality, a low capacity to appraise and reappraise reality and fantasy, or a high capacity to disguise the distortions. The disguises are accomplished by shifting meanings

and exaggerating and minimizing bits of reality as nidus for fantasy elabo-
ration" (p. 169). While this usually is an automatic cognitive information
processing style, nevertheless this tendency contributes to the perception
of the narcissistic person as deceitful, manipulative, and cunning.

In some narcissistic individuals, moral and value systems can be more
consistently relativistic or corrupt. They show disregard for conven-
tional values and society's rules through deceitful and dishonest behavior
(Akhtar, 1989; Cooper, 1998; Millon, 1998). Such behavior may range
from seductive, Don Juan-like recurrent efforts to conquer or passively
exploit others emotionally or financially, to conscious efforts to do the
"perfect crime," to actual crimes of revenge or to protect self-esteem or
status. However, narcissistic people who can present a variety of antisocial behavior are usually aware of moral norms and standards and able to
feel guilt and concern, but lack the capacity for deep commitment (O.
Kernberg, 1989a). Another expression of inconsistent superego pathology
stems from extremely harsh, constricting, and self-condemning attitudes
toward one's own assertiveness, achievements, and exhibitionistic strivings (Cooper, 1998). This type of superego dysregulation, often found in
the "shy" narcissistic personality, results in inhibiting self-scrutinizing and
self-shaming and feelings of inferiority and underachievement.

Malignant Narcissism

A more severe level of superego dysfunction in people with a narcissistic
personality structure has been captured by the term "malignant narcissism" (O. Kernberg, 1992, 1998a). This is a form of characterological
functioning that falls between NPD and ASPD, and it is characterized
by overt passive or active antisocial behavior, paranoid traits, and ego-
syntonic aggression and sadism that can be directed toward others as well
as toward the self. Kernberg suggests that malignant narcissism can be
expressed in seemingly self-justifiable violence, sadistic cruelty, or self-
destructiveness, where aggression and sadism is combined with elation
and increased self-esteem. It can also present as chronic suicidal preoccupation or ego-syntonic suicidal behavior attached to a fantasy that taking
one's life reflects superiority, control, and triumph over others as well
as over life and death. Maltsberger (1997) discussed examples of such
suicide that occur in a state of elated mood and omnipotent, thrill-seeking, grandiose ecstasy. In addition, manifestations of malignant narcissism
can involve sexual perversions where aggression and interpersonal sadism

interfuse with sexual desire and excitement. Such perverse behaviors are also characterized by non-differentiation or mixture of sexual aims, zones, organs, and gender. They replace sexual activities in the context of normal love, desire, and mutual intimacy, and are often a necessary condition for reaching sexual orgasm.

Kernberg (1998a) considered that people with malignant narcissism differ from people with ASPD since they still have capability for loyalty and concerns for others and for feeling guilty. He also noted that they have internalized "both aggressive and idealized superego precursors, leading to the idealization of the aggressive, sadistic features of the pathological grandiose self of these patients" (p. 375), and they indeed have the capacity to admire and depend upon sadistic and powerful people.

The expressions and severity of malignant narcissism depend on the predominance of self-righteous aggression and sadism, and on the degree to which aggression has infiltrated the pathological self-structure, that is, the extent to which self-esteem regulation relies upon self-righteous, aggressive, sadistic acts, and fantasies to maintain a sense of superiority. It also depends on the degree of superego dysregulation, that is, the balance between a non-aggressive value system with internalized idealized superego precursors and ego-ideals on the one hand, and primitive aggressive and sadistic superego precursors on the other (Kernberg, 1992).

Murder as an act of malignant narcissism has been studied by Stone (1989), who associated murderous feelings with the pain of being chronically humiliated or feeling like a nobody, or with the experience of being rejected and abruptly losing status. Malmquist (1996) described the dynamics of narcissistic killing as a righteous act of retaliation, a desperate effort to gain control, and to protect and raise self-esteem. Initial shame and withdrawal in response to humiliation may gradually trigger this urge for revenge, which is controlled over time by hatred, and enacted either internally as compulsive preoccupation or externally in the act of murder.

It is important to differentiate between (a) severe narcissistic reactions with aggressive, violent, or suicidal behavior emanating from inner experiences or interactions and life situations that are perceived as threatening to the individual's self-esteem, and (b) characterologically sustained malignant narcissism expressed as chronic intrapsychic and/or interpersonal ego-synthonic sadistic and paranoid attitudes and behavioral patterns that serve to buttress the regulation of self-esteem. The individual's ability to organize, plan, control, and experience joy or pleasure and peaks of high self-esteem constitutes another important dimension for evaluating and differentiating aggressive and malignant narcissistic behavior.

Case vignette

Mr. P, a successful professional, was in his early fifties when he finally decided to get married. Five months pregnant, his attractive wife unexpectedly and without prior discussion decided to have an abortion and move away to another part of the country. Devastated and deeply humiliated, Mr. P secretly began to develop a plan to kill her. Three years later he was invited to participate in a professional conference not far away from the city his former wife had moved to. During the conference he took a train to that city, went to the ex-wife's house and shot her, went back to the conference and led a discussion group later that afternoon. For the first time since his wife left, he noticed feeling calm and confident, and despite being prosecuted and serving prison time, he stated that he did not feel remorse.

Studies of political leadership have suggested that malignant narcissism can accompany grandiose ambitions and strivings for power and control in certain political dictators and tyrants. Glad (2002) found the malignant narcissistic syndrome most useful for describing and understanding the behavior of Josef Stalin, Adolph Hitler, and Saddam Hussein: "[T]he grandiosity, underlying sense of inferiority, the sadism, and the lack of scruples in dealing with perceived threats to their position . . . lack of genuine commitment to their comrades in arms and the values they espouse, as well as deep-seated proclivity to split the world in two, assigning all the darker traits of their own personalities to external enemies" (p. 22). The tyrants create an environment in which cruelty, paranoia, and criminal behavior become legitimized to reach and defend their grandiose, unlimited mission. The achievement of absolute power and control of their territories serve both to support the grandiose self through commanded acclaims and worship, and to eliminate critique and enemies, threats, and frustrations that can escalate their own inner conflicts and depression. On a personal level, both previous misdemeanors and present loneliness and self-doubts can easily be alleviated by surrounding supporters. The cycle of self-aggrandizement accompanied by increased success and power tends to escalate the tyrants' experiences of grandiose omnipotence and invulnerability which, in and by itself, can trigger paranoid control and hostility that gradually undermine their superior position.

Psychopathy, Antisocial Behavior, and Violence

The relatively high diagnostic overlap between NPD and ASPD (25%; Gunderson & Ronningstam, 2001) supports the view of a continuum ranging from pathological narcissism and NPD to malignant narcissism and ASPD (O. Kernberg, 1998a). Holdwick and colleagues (1998) found that NPD and ASPD share interpersonal exploitativeness, lack of empathy, and envy, and Blais, Hilsenroth, and Castlebury (1997) identified a sociopathic factor in NPD, lack of empathy, exploitation, envy, and grandiose sense of self-importance. Besides the more prototypic psychopathy with socially deviant behavior, Hare and colleagues (Harpur, Hakstian, & Hare, 1988; Hart & Hare, 1998) suggested that psychopathic symptomatology also involves a facet related to narcissism, called selfish, callous and remorseless use of others. It holds interpersonal and affective characteristics, such as egocentricity, superficiality, deceitfulness, callousness, and lack of remorse, empathy, and anxiety.

Studies of violence in social psychological and clinical research provide another connection between superego pathology and narcissism. Threats toward superior self-regard predicted aggressive and violent behavior (Baumeister et al., 1996), and NPD symptoms correlated with violence in adolescence and young adults (Johhnson et al., 2000). Nestor (2002) suggested that narcissistic personality traits are a clinical risk factor for violence. Narcissistic injury constitutes a specific pathway because it increases the risk for violent reactions, especially in psychopaths and people with antisocial conditions.

Of importance are the emotional and interpersonal sequels of moral and ethical dysregulation as they relate to self-esteem regulation in narcissistic people. Exploitative behavior, typical for both NPD and ASPD, may in narcissistic people be unconsciously motivated, a result of feeling superior or entitled, and serve to enhance self-image by gaining attention, admiration, and status. Exploitativeness can also stem from the narcissistic person having compromised empathy and being unable to identify the boundaries and feelings of others (Gunderson et al., 1991; Gunderson & Ronningstam, 2001; Ronningstam & Gunderson, 1990). In addition, NPD patients normally do not display recurrent antisocial behavior (except for those with advanced drug abuse who finance their addiction through regular criminal behavior), but they can occasionally commit criminal acts if enraged or as a means of avoiding defeat (Ronningstam & Gunderson, 1990).

Summary—The Psychopathic Narcissistic Personality Disorder

Obviously immoral or psychopathic behavior can also serve to protect or enhance the inflated self experience in narcissistic people. The sense of grandiosity is strongly related to feeling envious and entitled to exploit others. Disordered empathy, and aggressive, sadistic, revengeful behaviors are more pronounced, as is the specific superego pathology with lying, deceitful behavior. In summary, psychopathic NPD shares the following features with the arrogant type:

- Grandiose sense of self worth
- Exploitive behavior
- Envy
- Lack of commitment
- Impaired or lack of empathic capacity

Features exclusive for the psychopathic NPD type are:

- Irritability and raging reactions (Morey, Jones 1998)
- Callous and deceitful (Harpur, Hakstian, Hare 1988)
- Cunning/manipulative behavior (Harpur, et al., 1988)
- Lack of remorse or guilt (Harpur, et al., 1988)
- Interpersonal sadism (Kernberg, 1998a)
- Violent behavior (Baumeister, Smart, Boden, 1996)
- One or a few crimes (Gunderson, Ronningstam, 2001)

Other Determinants

Exclusion Criteria for NPD

The absence of overtly self-destructive behavior distinguishes NPD from BPD (Morey & Jones, 1998) because narcissistic patients normally do not involve themselves in self-harming and mutilating behavior or make manipulative suicide attempts. However, NPD patients may be involved in risk-taking behavior due to their belief in their own indestructibility or because of feeling superior when experiencing the thrill-seeking control of life over death. Feelings of emptiness are more predominant features of both BPD and ASPD because narcissistic people, due to their self-preoccupation, sense of superiority, and focus on achievements, tend to feel less emptiness (Ronningstam & Gunderson, 1990). Although patients with NPD can have corrupted consciences and commit one or a few crimes out of revenge or in response to threats to their self-esteem, the absence of a sustained pattern of antisocial behavior clearly differentiates narcissistic people from those with ASPD (Gunderson & Ronningstam, 2001).

Criteria for Long-term Stability

The reputation of NPD as being an unchangeable disorder and difficult to treat has been challenged both by new understanding of long-term changes in the personality and by new treatment modalities that have proven beneficial for patients with pathological narcissism. Nevertheless, the presence of two narcissistic characteristics—lack of commitment to others, and intense reactions to defeat and criticism from others—are associated with lack of improvement over time. In other words, the presence of these narcissistic problems is significantly associated with poor prognoses and absence of change and hence indicates more enduring forms of NPD (Ronningstam et al., 1995).

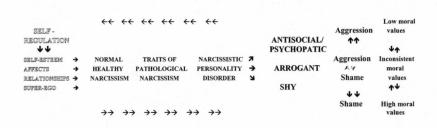

Figure 4.1. A dimensional regulatory model for narcissism – from normal narcissism to narcissistic personality disorder.

Conclusions

This chapter has outlined a dimensional diagnostic schema for identifying pathological narcissism and NPD. Both self-esteem dysregulation, the
core characteristic of narcissistic personalities, and affect dysregulation,
involving feelings of shame, anger, and envy, contribute to problems in
interpersonal relationships, leading to compromisd empathy and inability
to commit to others. Intense reactions to threats to self-esteem or to the
exaggerated self-image serve to protect the self-esteem, but such reactions
are also signs of affect dysregulation that cause problems in interpersonal
relations. The range of pathological narcissism, from predominant overt
aggression to proneness to shame and inhibition, reflects variations in
affect dysregulation that highly influence narcissistic individuals in managing both healthy and dysregulated aspects of their self-esteem. This
affect continuum together with the moral continuum differentiate the
arrogant NPD from both the shy narcissistic type and from antisocial and
psychopathic individuals (see figure 4.1).

5

Differentiating Pathological Narcissism

While it has been vital to identify discriminating features for each personality disorder, including NPD, to be able to differentiate them from each
other and from other mental illnesses, it has also proved to be of increasing clinical importance to identify the presence of pathological narcissism
in other mental conditions and disorders. Co-occurring narcissistic features can have major implications for course and prognosis, as well as for
the overall and in-depth understanding of the patient. Pathological narcissism can also have a major impact on the individual's experiences of and
attitudes toward treatment, and influence his or her motivation to engage
in a treatment alliance and comply with treatment recommendations,
even when the primary diagnosis is not a narcissistic disorder. The role of
major psychiatric symptoms, such as bulimia or anorexia, in narcissistic
self-esteem regulation is a relatively new avenue of inquiry (Steinberg &
Shaw, 1997). In addition, narcissistic symptoms in other disorders may
be overshadowed or erroneously attributed to other more predominant
symptoms (Simon, 2001). This chapter provides an overview of the clinical and empirical observations that can describe and explain some of
the specific interactions between NPD/pathological narcissism and near-
neighbor disorders and other major mental conditions.

The Interface with Axis II Personality Disorders

Patients who meet the *DSM* criteria for NPD more often than not also
meet criteria for other personality disorders. In fact, NPD is considered

to have one of the highest rates of diagnostic overlap among the Axis II disorders, and especially with disorders in the dramatic cluster (Gunderson, Ronningstam, & Smith, 1991; Morey & Jones 1998). Revisions of the NPD criteria in *DSM-IV* were aimed particularly at addressing this problem. The relationships between NPD and antisocial personality disorder (ASPD) and between NPD and borderline personality disorder (BPD) have received most theoretical and empirical attention, providing valuable and reliable differential diagnostic guidelines. In addition, people with histrionic personality disorder (HPD), obsessive-compulsive personality disorder (OCD), paranoid, and schizoid personality disorders can sometimes manifest narcissistic features, and vice versa. Seemingly similar and overlapping features may, however, have different intrapsychic and adaptive functions in different disorders, and the purpose with this overview is to specifically explore such differences.

NPD Versus ASPD and Psychopathy

Several authors and researchers have called attention to the relationship between NPD and ASPD (Gunderson, 1984; Livesley, Jackson, & Schroeder, 1992; Stone, 1993). O. Kernberg (1998a) suggested a spectrum of narcissistic pathology with antisocial behavior ranging from narcissistic personality, to the syndrome of malignant narcissism, to antisocial personality representing the most severe form of pathological narcissism. The antisocial person's more severe superego pathology involves lack of capacity for ethical self-regulation and compromised or absence of empathy and repudiation of others' moral and ethical dimensions; and lack of capacity for loyalty, guilt feelings, remorse, and concern for others. In contrast, the dynamics of the narcissistic individual involve defenses against unconscious envy with capacity to recognize good aspects in others, and their antisocial behaviors stem more from ego-syntonic entitlement and greed. As mentioned earlier (see chapter 4 this volume), the relatively high diagnostic overlap between ASPD and NPD (25%; Gunderson & Ronningstam, 2001) also reflects this relationship.

Other clinical differences between NPD and ASPD have also been identified. The presence of grandiosity in NPD and the antisocial individual's impaired capacity to be involved in mutual, nonexploitative relationships differentiate the two disorders. In addition, interpersonal manifestations and affective reactivity, especially rage reactions in response to criticism, are much more evident in NPD, while antisocial people show more acting out, particularly with drug and alcohol abuse, chronic unstable antisocial and criminal lifestyle, impulsivity, and sensation seeking (Gunderson & Ronningstam, 2001; Hart & Hare, 1998; Morey & Jones, 1998).

One study (Gunderson & Ronningstam, 2001) confirmed intrapsychic and interpersonal similarities between people with NPD and ASPD: Both have grandiose fantasies and believe in their invulnerability; both are in need of admiring attention, are entitled and envious, and have strong reactions to criticism. The major differences found in this study relate to narcissists being more grandiose—exaggerating their talents and feeling unique and superior—while people with ASPD are more actively exploitative and feel more empty. Both narcissistic and antisocial people are unempathic and exploitative. However, while antisocial peoples' ability to identify the needs and feelings of others relates to their aim and motivation (i.e., they can choose to ruthlessly ignore others or to empathize in the service of manipulation or exploitation), narcissistic people's empathic failures are due to an emotional or cognitive inability to identify with and feel for other people. Exploitativeness in antisocial patients is more likely to be consciously and actively related to materialistic or sexual gain, while exploitative behavior in narcissistic patients is more passive, or unwitting. More specifically, in people with NPD, exploitative behavior may be unconsciously motivated, a result of feeling superior or entitled and serving to enhance self-image by gaining attention, admiration, and status. Exploitativeness can also stem from the narcissistic person being unable to empathize and hence unable to identify the boundaries and feelings of others (Gunderson & Ronningstam, 2001; Gunderson et al., 1991). NPD patients normally do not display recurrent antisocial behavior (except for those with advanced drug abuse who finance their addiction through regular criminal behavior), but they can occasionally commit criminal acts if enraged or as a means of avoiding defeat (Ronningstam & Gunderson, 1990).

NPD and BPD

The relationship between NPD and BPD has received extensive attention (Adler, 1981; O. Kernberg, 1975; Masterson, 1981; see also chapter 1 this volume), and studies have previously reported substantial overlap between these disorders (Morey, 1988; Ronningstam & Gunderson, 1991). More recently, Holdwick, Hilsenroth, Castlebury, and Blais (1998) found that NPD shares with BPD affect dysregulation, impulsivity, and unstable relationships. Nevertheless, efforts to find a conceptual relativeness between NPD and BPD (see chapter 1 this volume) have resulted in both empirical and clinical evidence supporting their separateness. The most important discriminator is the inflated self-concept of NPD and its various manifestations of grandiosity, including exaggeration of talent, grandiose fantasies, and sense of uniqueness (Holdwick et al., 1998; Morey & Jones, 1998; Plakun, 1987; Ronningstam & Gunderson, 1991).

Akhtar (1992) identified the following structural and functional differences: the patient with NPD has a more cohesive self, with fewer tendencies to regressive fragmentation, whereas BPD patients have a more poorly integrated self with risk for the occurrence of psychotic-like states. Identity diffusion is manifest in BPD but masked in NPD. Due to the higher level of self-cohesiveness, NPD is associated with greater tolerance for aloneness and better work record, impulse control, and anxiety tolerance, while people with BPD, due to their lower level of cohesiveness, show more of self-mutilation and persistent rage. People with NPD are covertly shame ridden and insecure, and BPD patients have sustained identity diffusion and inferiority feelings. While narcissistic patients are less overtly self-destructive and less preoccupied with dependency and abandonment concerns (DSM-IV; Morey & Jones, 1998), they show more passive-aggressive features (Morey & Jones, 1998) and greater arrogance and haughtiness (Ronningstam & Gunderson, 1991). However, in response to severe humiliation, criticism, and defeat, people with NPD may react self-destructively with a controlled and calculated intention to kill themselves (Ronningstam & Maltsberger, 1998). This contrasts with BPD patients, whose self-destructive behavior is more impulsive and aimed at regaining caring attention (Gunderson, 2001). Both groups regard attention as important, but while borderlines seek nurturing attention because they need it, narcissists feel they deserve admiring attention because they consider themselves superior or exceptional (Ronningstam & Gunderson, 1991).

Recent extensive research efforts on identifying distinctive traits for borderline patients have improved discriminability of the BPD category in relation to other Axis II disorders, especially NPD. Zanarini, Gunderson, Frankenburg, and Chaunccey (1990) found the following features to be specific for BPD: quasi-psychotic thoughts, self-mutilation, manipulative suicide efforts, abandonment/engulfment/annihilation concerns, demandingness/entitlement, treatment regression, and countertransference difficulties. Gunderson (2001) suggested an integrated clinical synthesis for borderline patients consisting of intolerance of aloneness with impulsive behavior and lapses in reality testing as major reactions to separateness or abandonment. The corresponding traits for narcissistic patients would probably be intolerance of threats to the grandiose self-image and intense reactions, including protective cognitive and interpersonal maneuvers and feelings of rage and shame, in response to such threats. However, while the reactivity of people with BPD is more consistently manifest, the reactions of people with NPD may be expressed as overt anger, insecurity, or self-aggrandizing behavior but may also remain hidden and involve internal reactions and experiences without overt behaviors or reactions. In addition, studies of the pathogenesis of BPD have identified parental separations and losses, and experiences of sexual abuse as significant for the development of borderline pathology (Zanarini, 2000). These features together clearly demarcate BPD from NPD.

There are also notable similarities between NPD and BPD (Gunderson, 2001; Ronningstam & Gunderson, 1991): sensitivity to criticism, rage and entitlement, and reactions of anger to criticism. Entitled rage can be found in both NPD and BPD, but while this rage in people with NPD is triggered by threats to their superiority and to their sense of deserving special or inordinate rights, privileges, status and security, the entitled rage in people with BPD is triggered by their needs not being met and feelings of entitlement because of their suffering or victimization. It is very important to identify this type of rage because, when it is ignored, it tends to cause unproductive thriving on the patient's identification as defeated or victimized and prevents progress in treatment.

Similarly, patients with BPD can have narcissistic traits that influence the phenomenology of borderline symptoms. Self-destructive preoccupation in narcissistic BPD patients can be expressed in a particular combination of controlled, thrill-seeking or risk-taking self-destructive behavior that serves both to conquer inner feelings of badness as well as to maintain superior control. In other words, the narcissistic capacity for higher impulse control is attached to a borderline type of preoccupation with self-destructiveness, leading to a superior experience of balance between life and death, between control and destructiveness. As one patient described it, "I like to push myself to the edge, hold the razor blade so it touches the vein on my arm and imagine that I make deep bleeding cuts. In a peculiar way, the fact that I know I can cut myself, at the same time as I choose not to do so, makes me feel good, and I can be in this state for hours." Another patient with extensive knowledge on lethal dosages of various medications said, "I take exactly enough pills to 'knock myself out.' If I take one or two more there is a possibility that I will not wake up. Still, every time I hope I will die, and when I wake up I am disappointed that I did not die." For a third patient, a seemingly impulsive act of dramatic, severe self-harming behavior was actually well-planned and orchestrated and aimed solely toward a boyfriend who had decided to leave her. Afterward she felt calm, satisfied, triumphal, and done with the relationship. She considered the impulsive self-harming act a necessary vehicle toward her own independence.

Some patients with severe forms of NPD can actually function on a borderline level (O. Kernberg, 1998b) with lack of impulse control and anxiety tolerance and with severe chronic rage and paranoid ideations.

Pathological Narcissism and Other Personality Disorders

NPD and HPD   Both narcissistic and histrionic individuals tend to demonstrate exhibitionistic, dramatic, and seductive behavior. However, the histrionic person is capable of warmth, dependency, and genuine concern and commitment, while the narcissist is more cold, exploitative, manipulative, and aggressive (O. Kernberg, 1975; Millon, 1981; Morey & Jones, 1998). The histrionic person can appear spontaneous, without ulterior motives and seemingly sympathetic for all the trouble he or she causes, while the narcissistic individual is more controlled, calculating, and relentless.

NPD and Obsessive-Compulsive Personality Disorder (OCD)   Perfectionism is a common characteristic in both obsessive-compulsive and narcissistic patients (*DSM-IV*; Akhtar, 1989; Glickauf-Hughes & Wells, 1995; Rothstein, 1980; Sorotzkin, 1985;). People with either NPD or OCD may appear emotionally cold, with a strong need for control. Similar to histrionics but different from narcissists, however, the obsessive-compulsive person is capable of mutually deep relationships, intimacy, and commitments. Furthermore, OCD patients demonstrate considerable evidence of empathy and guilt, and their perfectionism is usually not accompanied by the devaluation, haughtiness, and demandingness found in narcissistic patients (Akhtar, 1989; O. Kernberg, 1975; Vaillant & Perry, 1980;).

While NPD people strive to *be* perfect and great, they are also preoccupied with the perfectionism and standards of others as a reflection of their own status and superiority. Obsessive-compulsives want to *do* things perfectly in order to be right, and perfectionism for such persons is related to mental and interpersonal control and to such high standards of their own performance that can cause self-inflicted distress and interference with vocational and social functioning. Perfectionist strivings in narcissistic individuals serve to avoid shame for not living up to grandiose standards, while in persons with OCD, perfectionism represents a need to avoid guilt for not meeting superego demands (Hewitt & Flett, 1991; Glickauf-Hughes & Wells, 1995). In addition, other-oriented perfectionism, that is, the unrealistic standards set up for others, has also been associated to narcissism. Evaluation of the perfectionism standards of others could involve both admiration and awe but, if not fulfilled, could also lead to blame, lack of trust, and feelings of hostility (Hewitt & Flett, 1991). The perfectionism attributed to or expected by the other serves to enhance the narcissistic person's own self-esteem.

Narcissistic characters with obsessive-compulsive features represent a specific diagnostic and treatment challenge (Glickauf-Hughes & Wells, 1995). These people have a more intellectually invested grandiose self-experience, and they want to obtain perfect knowledge, be intellectually superior, and have a sense of intellectual integrity. Obsessive-compulsive tendencies are defensively used in this mixed character to protect underlying narcissistic vulnerability, that is, unstable self-esteem, fragile sense of self, fear of being engulfed or used by others, and unconscious envy. Such people often feel unentitled to their feelings, and their relationships are characterized by ambivalence: While they feel they need relationships and are able to be more concerned and committed to others than people with NPD, they are also frightened by the risk of being engulfed, controlled, or mistreated by others.

NPD and Paranoid Personality Disorder   Both NPD and paranoid personalities display grandiose features. However, the paranoid person's grandiosity is usually connected to self-righteousness and self-justifying argumentation, and with anger that is unrelated to exploitativeness or envy (O. Kernberg, 1990). Narcissistic and paranoid individuals can also share devaluation, sensitivity to criticism, and lack of empathy (Akhtar, 1989). Narcissists are, however, more exploitative, envious, attention seeking, and arrogant. In addition, the narcissist is not pervasively mistrustful or in search of hidden motives. Narcissistic individuals sometimes show brief paranoid ideations, usually related to the belief that other people envy them and want to hurt them or counteract or spoil their achievements

(Ronningstam & Gunderson, 1990). Narcissistic personalities, function-ing on a lower level with malignant narcissism or borderline features (see above), can nevertheless manifest sustained paranoid features.

NPD and Schizoid Personality Disorder   Emotional aloofness and lack of mutual interpersonal relations or genuine deep interest in other people are common characteristics in both schizoid personality disorder and NPD. While narcissists are ambitious and high achieving, more actively in pursuit of advantageous or admiring relations, and more exploitative, schizoid individuals are passive, withdrawn, and resigned (Akhtar, 1989). However, in contrast to the narcissist, the schizoid individuals actually show a capacity to empathize with other people and to observe, describe, and evaluate others with depth and differentiation (O. Kernberg, 1990). In addition, a sense of superiority (Guntrip, 1969), inclinations toward a cognitive intellectual style (in contrast to an emotional, body-anchored style), and the presence of compensatory internal life and grandiose fan-tasies can also be found in both personality disorders. While narcissists can appear flamboyant and charming, the schizoid persons are indiffer-ent, colorless, and intangible.

The Interface with Axis I Disorders

The association between pathological narcissism and NPD and the major mental disorders has remained relatively unknown. This specific interface has actually received more attention in the psychoanalytic literature, in both theoretical and clinical in-depth studies of narcissistic patients with syndrome disorders. In most personality disorder studies the small samples of NPD have made it difficult to draw valid conclusions and empirically verify whether (a) NPD is primary and actually causing an accompanying Axis I disorder, or (b) NPD is secondary and an expression of a primary genetically or biologically based Axis I disorder; or (c) NPD is overlapping with an Axis I disorder and they have common etiological factors and/or an underlying predisposition of each other; or (d) NPD and the Axis I disorder actually are independent of each other. Studies of comorbidity of personality disorders and mental states in general, often including the effect of bi-axial diagnosis on treatment outcome, have shown very vari-able results (Tyrer, Gunderson, Lyons, & Tohen, 1997). The authors con-cluded that "the comorbid condition represents a heterogeneous group, in which the personality features can sometimes be used positively to aid outcome of treatment" (p. 254). A recent thought-provoking longitudinal study of the relationship of the near neighbor BPD to depressive disorder (Gunderson et. al, 2004) showed that although BPD and depressive disorder are sometimes independent of each other, more often the course of the depression could be predicted by the course of BPD, and improvement in BPD was often followed by improvement in depressive disorder, but not vice versa. In other words, it is more difficult to successfully treat an Axis I disorder, such as major depression, if a personality disorder such as BPD is present, and treatment of the Axis I disorder will not necessarily lead to improvement of the personality disorder.

Although the course and changes in the association between NPD in Axis I disorders still await longitudinal comparative studies, recent systematic conceptualization of pathological narcissism and NPD in terms of self-esteem regulation has helped identify associations with Axis I disorders as such symptoms often serve narcissistic functions in patients with co-occurring disorders. While self-regulation, patterns in interpersonal relationship, and capacity for empathy seem most relevant when differentiating NPD and narcissistic features in relation to other personality disorders, the understanding of self-serving or self-disrupting functions of specific symptoms, such as depression, mood elevation, anorexia and substance use, seem to signify the association between co-occurring narcissistic disorders and Axis I disorders.

NPD and Bipolar Spectrum Disorder

DSM-IV identifies grandiosity and inflated self-esteem as the most distinct feature both in NPD and in bipolar manic or hypomanic episodes. NPD is one of the most commonly occurring personality disorder among bipolar patients (Brieger, Ehrt, & Marneros, 2003), and bipolar disorder is the third most common Axis I disorder found in narcissistic patients (5–11%; see Ronningstam, 1996).

Several accounts in the clinical literature have outlined narcissistic characteristics in bipolar patients (see Ronningstam, 1996). Both Kohut (1971) and Morrison (1989) have described manic/hypomanic states in narcissistic patients. They also suggested that the self-regulatory functions are impaired in bipolar patients and that depression and mania can, for these patients, reflect a narcissistic balance that serves to direct feelings of rage and shame (Aleksandrowicz, 1980; Morrison, 1989).

Two major attempts to conceptualize this overlap have been made: from the bipolar spectrum, Akiskal (Akiskal, 1992; Akiskal & Mallya, 1987) introduced the hyperthymic temperament, and from a psycho-analytic perspective, Akhtar (1988) suggested a hypomanic personality disorder. People with hyperthymia bear several similarities with the narcissistic personality: being ambitious, high achieving, grandiose, boastful, exuberant, overoptimistic, self-assertive, and overconfident. They usually deny psychiatric symptoms but can have histories of brief episodes of depression, and they have been considered belonging to the bipolar spectrum mainly because of their strong family history of bipolar disorder. The hypomanic personality disorders share with narcissistic personalities the following features: grandiosity, self-absorption, social ease, articulateness, seductiveness, and moral, aesthetic, and vocational enthusiasm. However, contrary to people with NPD, hyperthymics are warm, people seeking, and meddlesome, and the hypomanics do not have the devaluating, secretly envious attitude of the narcissists or their seething vindictiveness and dedicated steadfast pursuit for perfectionism (Akhtar, 1988).

Our study (Stormberg, Ronningstam, Gunderson, & Tohen, 1998) found noteworthy similarities between the experiential, affective, and behavioral manifestations in both disorders in that bipolar patients in a hypomanic and acute manic phase actually exhibit most of the core characteristics for NPD: overt grandiosity, self-centeredness, entitlement, lack of empathy, arrogance, and boastful/pretentious behavior. Notable differences between narcissistic and bipolar disorders included the active search for admiring attention, devaluation of others, and secret profound envy of others found in narcissistic patients but not in patients with bipolar mania. We found no evidence of a narcissistic character structure or consistent features of pathological narcissism in bipolar patients when euthymic. In addition, hypomanics do not show contemptuous tendencies, and they lack the revengeful narcissistic rage and the extensive denial typical for narcissistic people (Akhtar, 1989).

As highlighted in the ongoing debate on the relationship between BPD and bipolar disorder (Dolan-Sewell et al., 2001), the criteria for overlapping personality disorders and bipolar disorder have different origins. While the grandiosity and inflated self-esteem in NPD patients is a long-term pervasive characterological pattern that is accompanied by intense reactions to perceived threats to the high self-regard, individuals with disorders within the bipolar spectrum have autonomous underlying mood shifts that cause temporary inflations in self-esteem. And while grandiosity in NPD is caused by a genetic predisposition (Torgersen et al., 2000) and a specific deformation in the personality structure, the grandiosity in bipolar disorder is generated by mood elevation caused by internal biological shifts. In narcissistic people, mood shifts usually occur in the context of external experiences that cause intense affective reactions. Feelings of shame, worthlessness, inferiority, or humiliation following events involving criticism, defeat, or loss of admiring support are prominent in depressed mood. Likewise, feelings of enthusiasm and excitement, confidence, and the grandiose self-experience evoked by intense admiring attention or involvement in competitive achievements and success accompany elevated mood. Nevertheless, despite these shifts in mood and affect, the underlying narcissistic personality structure with grandiosity and intense reactivity still remains relatively stable and unchanged, except in the event of a corrective life event (see chapter 8 this volume)

Narcissistic people with a comorbid bipolar spectrum disorder, that is, who have biological vulnerability and tend to have episodes of mood elevation or more consistent hyperthymia (Akiskal, 1992) or milder forms of mania, often report an ego-syntonic positive experience of such states. It may contribute to increased sense of capability and add to the individual's professional or creative capacity. Some people involved in exceptionally creative or intensely demanding professional activities actually consider their elevated mood a necessary condition for high job performance. A former successful CEO reported, "I needed to multitask and manage at a very high pace during a 10–15 hour work day, and I totally depended upon my elevated mood to succeed in my work." And a professor in music said, "I like my hypomanic state because it stimulates my creativity and I am able to compose and write well." Sudden mood change, that is, decrease in elevation or onset of depression, may for such people have devastating consequences, leading to career interruption, loss of creative capability, and long-term inability to perform professionally. A positive attitude to mood elevation can also decrease motivation for long-term mood-stabilizing treatment because such treatment may intensify inner experiences of inferiority and limitations. This is in contrast to those narcissistic people for whom inner emotional and intellectual control is essential for the sense of superiority. Such people usually dread the challenging intrusion of mood elevation because they fear to loose a sense of inner mastery and control.

It is reasonable to conclude that hyperthymia/hypomania/mood elevation and pathological narcissism are conceptually and phenomenologically different. Following Vaglum's (1999) approach to the relationship between NPD and substance abuse (see below), it also seems appropriate to propose an interactive model for co-occurring pathological narcissism/ NPD and the bipolar spectrum disorders. Narcissistically invested events and experiences can evoke and influence mood swings and mood swings can have a major impact on narcissistic self-esteem and affect regulation. Of interest is what factors make some but not all NPD patients become bipolar or vice versa, and what makes some bipolar patients maintain enduring pathological narcissism. Notable is the bipolar NPD patients' appreciation for mood elevation and capability to integrate high energy and activity level into periods of successful personality functioning, and even highly valuable professional or creative achievements. In these patients we find a strong positive covariation between both healthy and pathological aspects of narcissism and one side of the bipolarity elevated mood. Identifying the presence of genetic or biological communalities awaits further research.

NPD and Depressive Disorder and Dysthymia

Acute depression as a reaction to severe narcissistic humiliation, defeats, failures, or losses, often in combination with suicidal ideations, usually forces the normally symptom-free narcissistic patient to psychiatric treatment. Depression in such patients usually occurs in the context of a failure in the self-regulatory processes that support the pathological grandiose self. In other words, depression can be seen as an effect of decreased self-esteem and a consequence of the depleted or depreciated self in narcissistic patient (O. Kernberg, 1975; Kohut, 1977). Because feeling of shame is the active response to such failures and depletion of ideals, Morrison (1989) consider depression in narcissistic people as secondary to underlying shame. This type of depression, often called "empty depression," is characterized by "guiltless despair," feelings of emptiness and depletion, hopelessness, meaninglessness, and lethargy (Kohut, 1977). Self-pity can accompany a depressive reaction in response to narcissistic injury, humiliation, or empathic failure. In chronic empty depression, self-pity, often accompanied by self-righteousness and complaints toward the person causing the humiliation, may indicate an effort to maintain self-cohesion (S. Wilson, 1985). Other types of depression or depressive reactions may be caused by a loss of control or loss of a sense of mastery or status. Such depression is distinguished by irritability and feelings of helplessness, worthlessness, envy, and impotent rage. Dysthymia, a chronic state of boredom, aloneness, stimulus hunger, dissatisfaction, and feelings of meaninglessness, is a reaction to unavoidable gradual self-disillusion and repeated failures in narcissistic individuals (Millon, 1981).

A specific type of depression occurs more frequently and intensely in midlife when the narcissistic individual is confronted with aging and life's inevitable limitations (O. Kernberg, 1980). The mourning over lost gratifications or narcissistically invested functions or material supplies, and the painful awareness of aloneness and the consequences of one's own narcissistically geared actions and choices, can cause a chronic pattern of devaluation, denial, pessimism, bitterness, and resentment. Such depression may make the narcissistic patient more motivated for treatment and changes. However, there is also a potential for suicide in those for whom changes seem less of a possibility or for whom the experience of morning and guilt is intolerable. Kernberg considered the capacity for tolerance of depression and mourning to be an indication for improved prognosis in narcissistic patients, especially if the depression is accompanied by guilt, regret, and concern.

One complexity in narcissistic patients may paradoxically be the absence of overt depressive symptoms. Because of low affect tolerance, such patients make various efforts to escape intolerable feelings such as rage and shame, hopelessness, and experiences of limitations. Suicidal ideations and behavior in narcissistic patients may occur in the absence of depression (O. Kernberg, 1992; Maltsberger, 1998; see chapter 7 this volume). Other types of defensive attitudes, cults or ideologies, or constrictive lifestyles may also protect against narcissistic failure and replace a course toward severe depression in midlife or later (O. Kernberg, 1980).

Major depression and dysthymia are the most common concomitant Axis I disorders in patients with NPD (42–50%). Studies of the opposite interrelation, that is, the presence of NPD in major depression, have earlier shown much lower prevalence rates (0–5%; see Ronningstam, 1996). However, more recent empirical studies of major depression in personality disorders by Fava and colleagues found higher prevalence rates for NPD (8.1–16.4%). They found NPD and several other personality disorders to be more common in depression with anger attacks than without such attacks (Fava & Rosenbaum, 1998; Tedlow et al., 1999), and significantly more common in early-onset major depression (Fava et al., 1996). They also noticed instability in personality disorder diagnosis. Following an 8-week fluoxetine treatment, there was a significant reduction both in the number of patients meeting criteria for NPD (and eight other personality disorders) and in the mean number of NPD criteria found among the narcissistic patients. Decrease in the number of criteria met for NPD was significantly related to improvement in depressive symptoms (Fava et al., 2002). These results are interesting and notable because they contradict some of the previous clinical observations on depression in narcissistic patients, that is, of a temporary decrease in major narcissistic traits, such as grandiosity, in acutely depressed narcissistic patients (Ronningstam, Gunderson, & Lyons, 1995) and increased NPD rates in patients with remitted depression (Joffe & Regan, 1988). In addition, the previously noted treatment resistant depression in NPD patients was also challenged by Fava and colleague's studies. These different observations indicate a complexity of co-occurring pathological narcissism and depression. This also points to an important avenue for further longitudinal explorations of the role of narcissistic personality functioning in depression, in particular, reactive depression and depression due to chronic inner massive self-criticism or self-hatred.

People who have encountered severe narcissistic threats and humiliation through interrupted careers (Ronningstam & Anick, 2001) can show an unusual complexity in their experience of depression related to loss of their former professional affiliation and working capacity. Although such depression can be manageable via a psychopharmacological treatment modality, a major aspect of these people's depression seemed related to unresolved feelings about their career interruption and continuing professional failures. These feelings included emptiness, inadequacy, humiliation, rage, shame, envy, and worthlessness (see chapter 6 this volume).

NPD, Addiction, and Substance-use Disorders

Narcissistic vulnerability, impulse dysregulation, and affect intolerance in the development of drug abuse and dependency have been considered important predisposing factors in substance abuse disorders (Vaillant, 1988; Richman, Flaherty, & Rosendale, 1996), and the presence of NPD has actually been considered a risk factor for the development of cocaine abuse (Yates, Fulton, Gabel, & Brass, 1989).

Psychoanalytic studies noted the function of substance abuse as an important defensive action to protect narcissistic vulnerability. Wurmser (1974) suggested that an overwhelming narcissistic crisis is the specific cause of the manifestation of addictive illness: "an actualization of a life-long massive conflict about omnipotence and grandiosity, meaning and trust" (p. 826), accompanied by feelings of disillusionment, rage, depression, and anxiety. The addiction is an attempt to reestablish lost omnipotence and grandiosity, or it can be used as a defense against intolerable feelings of rage, shame, and depression. O. Kernberg (1975) wrote: "In the case of narcissistic personalities, alcohol and drug intake may constitute a predominant mechanism to 'refuel' the pathological grandiose self and assure its omnipotence and protection against a potentially frustrating and hostile environment in which gratification and admiration are not forthcoming" (p. 222). Khantzian (1980, 1982, 1985) considered narcotics to be used for self-medication purposes to diminish the regressive and disorganizing influence of intense rage and aggression on the ego. In other words, these accounts acknowledge the adaptive function of drug use for compensating narcissistic vulnerability and self-esteem fluctuations, for maintaining self-control and mastery of impulses and affects, and for self-protection and strengthening boundaries between the internal and external world.

Dodes (1990) identified the narcissistic impairment in addicts as a vulnerability to experiences of powerlessness. He highlighted the role of rage as an impelling drive behind addictive behavior, triggered by a loss of power and control over one's affects and mind. He suggested that addiction helps maintaining omnipotence and control over one's own affective states to avoid the experience of helplessness caused by overwhelming affects and psychic trauma. He also believed drug use to be a tool that serves to re-establish omnipotence and control, leading to a corrective experience in which individuals take control of their affective states.

Of specific relevance are the narcissistic effects of different substances. Cocaine and other stimulants produce a sense of mastery, control, and grandeur that increases self-esteem and frustration tolerance and a sense of self-sufficiency. Opiates and barbiturates influence affect regulation and reduce feelings of shame, rage, emptiness, and worthlessness. Psychedelic drugs may contribute to an experience of boundlessness and expansive and illusional grandiosity (Khantzian, 1979; Wurmser, 1974). With regard to alcohol, Tähkä (1979) suggested that the relation between pathological narcissism and alcoholism follows a path of narcissistic regression. Different mental approaches for maintaining self-esteem are developed during the course of alcoholism, with increased dependence upon compensatory external self-objects at more severe levels of the illness.

Although a relatively low rate of substance abusers seeking treatment fulfill the criteria for NPD (7%), many do indeed report a high prevalence of narcissistic traits (Vaglum, 1999), and substance use disorder was indeed the second most frequently concomitant Axis I disorder in NPD patients (24–50%; see Ronningstam, 1996). Empirical studies reporting on personality disorders in alcohol and substance abuse disorders indicate relatively high rates of NPD for drug abusers (12–38%) and lower rates for alcohol abusers (6–7%; see Ronningstam, 1996). Yates et al. (1989) suggested that cocaine abusers are more likely than non-cocaine abusers to display NPD traits, and they actually consider NPD to be a risk factor for the development of cocaine abuse. Vaglum (1999) concluded that although narcissistic traits and NPD seem unrelated to the further course of addiction, NPD may increase the risk of becoming an addict and may contribute to medical disorders and death among addicts due to risk taking and lack of self-care. Of interest is what factors make some but not all NPD patients become drug abusers. Identification of the presence of genetic or biological communalities awaits further research. Differences in superego functioning or proneness to dependency or addiction in the underlying character functions may play a role. However, most evidence seems to suggest that more severe forms of affect intolerance, self-esteem instability, or exceptional susceptibility to grandiose self-experience can make some narcissistic patients more prone to drug abuse.

NPD and Eating Disorders

Weight and body shape are substantially related to self-esteem in people with eating disorders. They usually consider weight loss a major achievement and indication of extraordinary self-discipline, and weight-gain a sign of failure of self-control (*DSM-IV*). Earlier clinical literature described more specific narcissistic tendencies in patients with anorexia, such as narcissistic denial of reality, moral pride, and sense of having been "unconsciously chosen" within their families (P. Wilson, 1983). In addition, anorexic patients had omnipotent fantasies and a grandiose sense of superiority in areas of intelligence, morality, and control, accompanied by feelings of contempt and expressions of underlying narcissistic rage (Hogan 1983a, 1983b, 1983c). Anorexia was associated with self-esteem and self-control (Sours, 1974), and Goodsitt (1985) outlined several nar-

cissistic features as evidence of the anorexic patient's incapacity to maintain internal self-esteem: grandiosity, exhibitionism, reactivity, power,
and control. Self-esteem is restored through control of ingestion and the
body-self. C. Johnson and Connors (1987) suggested two character disorders in patients with eating disorders: borderline and false self/narcis-
sistic. A person with the latter disorder presents attempts to "compensate
for or hide interoceptive deficits," and is considered to have greater ego
resources than the borderline type. Feelings of shame have been associated with self-esteem specifically in anorexic patients. They tend to link
self-experience to body shape and to ineffective self-regulation, and a
sense of incompetence with vulnerability to external control. Eating-asso-
ciated shame was considered a consequence of eating-disordered behavior
and the strongest predictor of the severity of eating disorder symptoms
(Burney & Irwin, 2000).

Empirical studies on both anorexia and bulimia have supported these
observations and reported on self-esteem regulation, perfectionism,
increased self-criticism, and interpersonal hypersensitivity in patients
with eating disorders (Steiger, Gauvin, & Jabalpurwala, 1999; Steiger,
Jabalpurwala, Champagne, & Stotland, 1997; Steinberg & Shaw, 1997).
Studies reporting on personality disorders in eating disorders have shown
inconsistent results, with NPD rates varying from 0% to 33% (see Ronningstam, 1996). One study on the presence of pathological narcissism
in anorexic subjects (Ronningstam, 1992) showed that anorexics (both
restricted and bulimic type) share with patients diagnosed as NPD an
unrealistic sense of uniqueness and superiority, and a preoccupation with
others' envy. However, while narcissists usually feel superior or unique
because of their special talents, extraordinary intelligence or sensitivity,
or exceptional and exquisite taste, anorexics feel unique because of their
involvement in the starving process and the accompanying special personal lifestyle. The anorexics feel superior because of their capacity for
extreme weight loss, their ability to control their emotions, and their need
for food and body weight. They also feel superior because they do not
need what other people need in terms of food and attention. They disdain people who "live a normal life, and are fat and lazy." While anorexics
consider their low body weight and capacity to control their lifestyle to
be the reasons for others' envy, narcissists believe they are envied because
of their uniqueness and their talents, success, or achievements (Ronningstam, 1992).

Pathological Narcissism in Trauma and Posttraumatic Stress Disorder

Preexisting NPD is likely to heighten sensitivity to trauma and enhance vulnerability to stress at lower levels of trauma. In addition, the symptoms of posttraumatic stress disorder (PTSD) may present differently in people with NPD. War veterans with narcissistic character and PTSD showed a tendency to use trauma symptoms as a mechanism to increase self-esteem. W. Johnson (1995) suggested that "the narcissistic personality with a profound need for the advantage of 'warrior status' may be more vulnerable to psychic trauma and may subsequently perpetuate falsehoods to account for their experience and bolster a fragile sense of self" (p. 41). The use of PTSD symptoms for narcissistic self-esteem regulation as compared to the regular presentation of PTSD is an important differential diagnostic feature to consider in treatment planning.

Trauma-associated narcissistic symptoms (TANS; Simon, 2001; see above)—narcissistic reactions and symptoms associated with an external traumatically stressful experience or event—have several features in common with PTSD. Both may share anxiety, avoidance, and depression, as well as feelings of shame and humiliation. However, while PTSD symptoms relate to trauma involving threats to physical survival and safety, TANS can be triggered by different, usually interpersonal, traumatic stressors that can vary in both intensity and duration but nevertheless can be experienced as a narcissistic humiliation, attack, or trauma. PTSD is an anxiety disorder, whereas TANS is related to a character disorder with underlying pathological narcissism or NPD, and the course of PTSD is more chronic, whereas TANS may subside rather fast, persist over time, or, in severe cases with exacerbating NPD, develop into a long-term disabling condition.

NPD and Anxiety and Panic Disorders

Narcissistic pathology and anxiety disorders have seldom been commented on in clinical literature. Overall very low NPD rates (0–5%) were found in studies reporting on personality disorders in anxiety and panic disorders, and acutely ill panic disorder patients score lower NPD rates (see Ronningstam, 1996). The only account on panic and anxiety reactions related to problems with self-esteem regulation described patients suffering from stage fright (Gabbard, 1979, 1983, 1997; see also chapter 6 this volume).

NPD and Paranoid Psychosis or Schizophrenia with Grandiose Delusions

Although grandiosity occurs in both NPD and psychotic disorders or schizophrenia, the presence of psychotic illness and loss of reality testing contraindicate a diagnosis of NPD (O. Kernberg, 1990). Nevertheless, experiences of severe narcissistic disillusionment can without necessary support develop into worsening narcissistic psychopathology (Ronningstam et al., 1995), which in severe cases may include specific grandiose delusions or paranoid revengeful reactions. Millon (1996) describes the tendency of narcissistic people to decompensate into paranoid disorders after experiences of serious failure, betrayal, or humiliation. They may "isolate themselves from the corrective effects of shared thinking" (p. 414) and devote themselves to compensatory grandiosity, jealousy, or persecutory delusions and verbal self-righteous tirades toward those who have failed to acknowledge their superiority. *DSM-IV* also acknowledges the grandiose type of delusional disorder when "the central theme of the delusion is the conviction of having some great (but unrecognized) talent or insight or having made some important discovery" (p. 297). Less common is the idea of having a special identity or being affiliated to a famous person.

Pathological Narcissism and Nonverbal Learning Disorder

Nonverbal learning disabilities, a right hemispheric dysfunction that leads to deficits in social skills and capacity to understand the social environment and recognize nonverbal cues, is a relatively unexplored area of interface with pathological narcissism and self-esteem regulation. The impairment in social-emotional processing involves missing out on nonverbal aspects of language and difficulties understanding subtleties in others' emotions and experiences of social distress when interacting with other people. It also includes impaired perception and imaginary functions that lead to difficulties in understanding the social environment, and to distortion of perceptual experience and limitations in inner psychological experiences and adaptive behavior (Semrud-Clikeman & Hynd, 1990). Garber (1989,

1991) noted that learning disabilities in children are associated with a deficit in empathy causing serious difficulties in social relationships. Children with such deficit are unable to understand the impact of their own actions and interactive behavior, while being themselves overly sensitive to emotional slights and hurts from others.

Although Asperger's syndrome, another subtype of nonverbal learning disabilities, has been associated with schizoid personality disorder (Tantam, 1988; Wolff, 1995), several accounts also report on typical narcissistic characteristics in people with Asperger's syndrome. Those include perfectionism and impaired capacity for empathy (Attwood, 1998), life-long eccentricity (Tantam, 1988), and a general lack of social and emotional reciprocity (DSM-IV). People with Asperger's syndrome usually have good intellectual functioning in specific areas, such as capacity for recalling information, defining words, and visual thinking. They may even be remarkably intelligent, despite weaknesses in comprehension and problem solving, and outstanding contributions within science and art have been attributable to people with Asperger's syndrome (Attwood, 1998).

The co-occurrence of these specific neurological dysfunctions and narcissistic traits needs further study. The main area of inquiry is how impaired intersubjectivity, impaired empathy, and self-esteem dysregulation with compensatory strategies used for covering an inner sense of incapacity and vague defectiveness interact with the development of pathological narcissism and NPD. Differentiating the possible co-occurrence of nonverbal learning disorder, or a possible neurological cause of impaired capacity for empathy, from characterological interpersonal problems with insensitivity, misunderstanding and impaired empathy, is absultely crucial and of major clinical importance for understanding the patient and for treatment planning and making appropriate therapeutic interventions.

Somatization and Hypochondriasis

Cooper (1998) identified hypochondrias as the somatic expression of a core weakness of the self-representations of the body in narcissistic individuals, and Krystal (1998) stated that "psychosomatic illness can be considered as one of the most solid and dependable 'protections' against the recognition of narcissistic defects and inadequacies in object relations (i.e., the consequences of severe narcissistic injuries)" (p. 312). Alexithymia, that is, impaired ability to name and localize emotions and find feelings useful for information processing and for personal motivation, decision making, and pursuits, is a central feature in severe affect dysregulation (see chapter 4 this volume). Affect regression combined with alexithymia makes the individual vulnerable to the collapse of the normal psychophysiological interactive functions of affect signals, which leads to somatization. In the interface between self-esteem and affect dysregulation and somatic symptoms/conditions, it is very important to differentiate between (a) affect regression into actual or exaggerated experiences of somatic symptoms due to an inability to tolerate intense affects evoked by narcissistic challenges or threats in real life; and (b) narcissistic gains related to actual or exaggerated experiences of somatic symptoms/conditions, that is, systematic retreat into a somatic condition to protect and increase self-esteem, ward off narcissistic challenges, or even to gain attention, admiration, and special treatment.

Conclusions

This chapter has described the broad interface between pathological narcissism and other mental disorders. The fact that pathological narcissism co-occurs with numerous other mental states and disorders supports a dimensional model for narcissism in terms of self-esteem, affect, and interpersonal regulation (see figure 4.1 and table 4.1 this volume). Of special importance when distinguishing pathological narcissism and NPD in other conditions is to identify the narcissistic meaning and regulatory function of a specific mental characteristic or symptom. Focusing on understanding self-esteem regulation and exploring the self-regulatory and interpersonal meaning of a symptom, attitude, or behavior can be helpful and sometimes even crucial in the evaluation and treatment of narcissistic people and with people who present other major conditions with accompanying narcissistic pathology.

6

Asset or Disruption?

Narcissism in the Workplace

Narcissistic Aspects of Work

Vocational activities and professional careers are usually associated with healthy narcissistic investment. For most people, the capacity to work—that is, to create, produce, collaborate, accomplish, achieve, and succeed—is a source of personal pride and satisfaction. The meaning of work and its impact on an individual's self-esteem are a relatively new topic of clinical investigation. Axelrod (1999) noted that, "[i]n adulthood, the ego ideal is, in part, a repository of images and fantasies associated with successful working . . . The fuller articulation of coherent, realistic, yet highly personal ideals is an important part of all work-related interventions and has significant benefits for self-esteem" (p. 11). Levine (1997) identified work as an arena for self-esteem regulation and ego identity and for definition of the self. Kohut (1977) suggested that an integration of ambition and guiding ideals into meaningful goal-oriented work contributes to increased self-cohesiveness and psychological health. He also pointed out that good work could improve shattered self-esteem. Work has long been considered an essential part of psychiatric rehabilitation. Recent studies have pointed to the importance of work for life quality and self-esteem in psychiatrically disabled people. Van Dongen (1996) found that work provided distraction from symptoms and contributed to better mental health. Arns and Linney (1993) reported that improvement in vocational status resulted in higher self-efficacy, self-esteem, and life satisfaction.

The workforce is also the arena for exceptional narcissistic accomplishments. Charisma, self-confidence, foresight, assertiveness, and capacity to personify ideals, visions, and changes are personality qualities that we find among those leaders who dominate the modern business and political world. According to Maccoby (2000), narcissistic leaders "are innovators, driven in business to gain power and glory. Productive narcissists are experts in their industries, but they go beyond it. They also pose the critical questions. They want to learn everything about everything that affects the company and its products. Unlike erotics, they want to be admired not loved. And unlike obsessives, they are not troubled by their superego so they are able to aggressively pursue their goals" (p. 72). They also understand the vision, that is, to combine the uncombinable and to see the yet-to-be-seen, and with their "personal magnetism" they can inspire and activate people, attract followers, and achieve remarkable results. However, as Maccoby also mentioned, the danger with narcissistic leaders is that they depend upon others for admiration and adulation, and that "faults tend to become even more pronounced as he becomes more successful" (p. 73). Difficulties with learning and listening to others, sensitivity to criticism, self-righteousness, lack of empathy, extreme need for independence, inability to mentor, and a desire for ruthless competition make narcissistic leaders vulnerable. Tendencies to expansive grandiosity, excessive risk taking, paranoid ideations, and isolation usually lead to leadership collapse. O. Kernberg (1998c) described a more severely disturbed type of narcissistic leadership characterized by corruptive behavior and primitive personality functioning. This leader, who is strongly power motivated, consciously exploits the organization and feels entitled to use the position for multiple personal need gratifications. Tendencies to splitting both within and outside the organization, identifying enemies that justify dishonest or even antisocial actions, and escalation of control associated with paranoid suspiciousness are a few of the noticeable markers for this leadership development (see chapter 4 this volume).

However, in other areas, such as art, music, film, and literature, exceptional personalities have designed space for themselves that grants the full range of their exhibitionistic creativity as well as narcissistic eccentricity. The exceptionally ingenious and outlandish Spanish artist Salvador Dali not only integrated the Narcissus myth in his painting *Metamorphosis of Narcissus* and poetry, "The Metamorphosis of Narcissus" (1937), using a self-created "paranoiac-critical method," but he also struggled with narcissistic self-absorption, intense feelings of shame, and a tormenting fear of homosexuality (Gibson, 1997). Ingmar Bergman, the equally eccentric and creative Swedish film maker, has had a remarkable capacity to project his inner personal dynamics onto the screen in ways that could be appreciated by audiences all over the world. His life-long problems with intimacy and relationships and his sharp oscillations between exceptionally aggrandizing and severely humiliating experiences have been thoroughly documented (Bergman, 1987; Ullman, 1976). Both of these artists created their own space. Bergman chose Fårö, a small island in the Baltic Sea, as his personal compound and site for much of his stage production. The unique theater-museum Fundacio Gala-Salvador Dali, in Figueres, Catalonia, Spain, is the ultimate expressive account of Dali's imaginative creativity.

Arshile Gorky, the Armenian-American artist who received much recognition after his premature death, represents yet another example of a person with exceptional talent and creativity with narcissistic vicissitudes. Having personally experienced the traumatic events of the Armenian genocide in his home town, the city of Van, he came to the United States with an inner conviction that he owned the potential to become an outstanding artist. Once in the United States, he transformed himself from a penniless immigrant by borrowing a new identity as an artist. He developed a confident and exaggerated personal style to accentuate his ideas and fantasies about being a painter, that is, "the lonely artist pitting himself against the world antagonism" (Spender, 1999, p. 63). In other words, he created an image of himself as "the distinguished artist," an image that he worked hard to live up to. Exposed to the world's masterpieces, which he meticulously studied in awe, he developed his own ability for artistic expressions, and soon he was totally immersed in his artwork. Initially he imitated and borrowed the techniques of other masters, and he was known to draw like Sargent and paint like Rembrandt, Cézanne, and Picasso. Soon, however, Gorky's own exceptional creative talents became obvious to his teachers and peers. Indeed, he was in the vanguard of the American modern art and developed a remarkable mature originality in his pioneering abstract expressionistic work. Those more intimate with him witnessed another side, a man who had no sense of the other person and a very limited capacity for understanding and empathizing with others. Torn between possessiveness, jealousy, and violence, he wanted to control those close to him, and his passionate love turned into efforts to mold the other into someone or something that fit his liking. Although Gorky gained artistic reputation and succeeded extremely well during his short life, it was not until after his tragic death by suicide that his works were fully appreciated and achieved international recognition. He finally gained in death the position among the masters that he so eagerly had aspired to in life.

The Challenge of Getting Along

The workplace may present extraordinary challenges for the narcissistic individual as it usually requires a capacity to understand and attend to more or less explicit rules for and patterns of interpersonal interactions. The team belongingness among peer colleagues, the hierarchical interaction vis-à-vis supervisors, managers, and bosses/leaders and the relationship with partners outside the workplace can contribute to difficult internal experiences and interpersonal conflicts for narcissistic people. Power, competition, sub-group belongingness, informal hierarchies of status and popularity, gossip, and so on, can trigger unmanageable rage and/or insecurity. Despite exceptional skills and knowledge, it is not uncommon that these interpersonal conditions create such overwhelming problems for the narcissistic person, often expressed in an inability or unwillingness to collaborate and follow rules for communication and exchange, rage outbursts, ignoring or deliberately overstepping rules and boundaries, effort to dominate and take control, or to form special or influential relationships. The person may struggle with experiences of being outside, excluded, or isolated, or with feelings of insecurity, envy, or resentment toward more senior or competent people, or with issues related to specialness and advantages.

Case Vignette

Mr K, a skilled financial analyst, was hired by a progressive, fast-growing company to develop a specific long-term project. Chosen by the president and positioned to report directly to him, Mr. K immediately encountered certain reactions from different groups of staff in the company. Being arrogant and forceful, Mr. K soon found that some colleagues had began to resent him and that they excluded him from some of the social interactions at lunchtime. Moreover, he found that when he needed to collaborate with colleagues from the company's regular analyst group, they tended to create difficulties, which triggered Mr. K's frustration and anger. Despite being exceptionally knowledgeable and able to develop a very successful and most profitable project and despite his special relationship to the boss who was immensely satisfied with his work, Mr. K still felt isolated from the rest of the company and extremely frustrated with some of his colleagues. As time went on, his conflicts with different people both within and outside the company just escalated. Three years later Mr. K was fired the day after he had received the company's excellence award; the reason given was his lack of interpersonal skills and flexibility.

The Necessary Niche in the Workplace

Narcissistic people often present a puzzle because they can be highly creative and accomplished and yet highly constrained by their specific personality limitations. The capacity for work may represent a narrow line between passive paranoid withdrawal and exceptional ability, and some people work best when their workplace is like a secluded niche, where they can engage in solitary activity with minimal interactions.

Case vignette

Ms. H, a matter-of-fact woman in her late forties, who preferred structure, control, and solitude, had managed exceptionally well in her professional career as a computer consultant. Due to her highly specialized and unusually well-defined area of expertise, she had been contracted by several companies that relied entirely upon her services. Being remarkably capable of solving "the most impossible problems" and adjusting to the increasing demands of fast-developing companies, Ms. H was highly regarded and well paid. During the more than 20 years she had consulted for these companies, she had learned to dictate her conditions, that is, set her own hours and demand her own solitary office space with specific interior conditions, and she was used to having all her requirements met. Ms. H certainly came across as superior, self-centered, eccentric, and somewhat arrogant; she was intolerant of others' limitations and often sarcastic and mocking toward others' incompetence and lack of knowledge. Ms. H did not hide the fact that she was uncomfortable with people, and she spent most of her time outside work alone. Having grown up in a wealthy family with an alcoholic mother and a hardworking, distant father, she struggled with anger and resentment. She sensed that she had survived by prematurely developing a cynical, superior attitude, and a capacity for observing others, which had helped protect her from what she considered the pathetic stupidity and ignorance of her parent. On the other hand, she also knew that she was smart and that she had a success-oriented side to her personality along with a gradually developing capacity of communicating with others through her professional activities.

Counterproductive Work Behavior

The interface between narcissism and work is multifaceted, and the work arena can also be the site for unhealthy and even severely pathological narcissistic behavior. These involve both individual, dyadic and group and systemic/organizational interactions that can be more or less destructive to the working environment and to individual and organizational productivity. The first study to include narcissism as an aspect of counterproductive work behavior (Penney & Spector, 2002) focused on the relationship between threatened egotism and aggression in the workplace. Counterproductive work behavior that previously has been associated with personality characteristics such as Machiavellianism and agreeableness involves such acts as theft, sabotage, interpersonal aggression, and spreading rumors. An assumption of the study was that personality variables that are related to aggressive behavior in general would also be related to workplace aggression. This is in line with recent research on self-esteem and threatened egotism (see chapter 4 this volume), which shows that people with high but unstable self-esteem and an inflated self-image react with aggressive or hostile behavior to threats to their egos (Bushman & Baumeister, 1998). The results from Penney and Spector (2002) showed that narcissistic people more frequently experienced anger and expressed their anger by engaging in counterproductive work behavior, especially under conditions with high job constraints (e.g., constraints in equipment, supplies, budget, task preparations, time availability, orwork environment). They also found that narcissistic people were more likely to perceive job constraints and react to them intensively. On the other hand, sometimes equally detrimental for workplace ethics is the tendency found in highly narcissistic people to base their motivation for work on perceived self-enhancement opportunities for themselves (Wallace & Baumeister, 2002). Work performance for such people is more a matter of seeking admiration and opportunities for personal success than to conform to team efforts and corporate goals, and may even in certain cases lead to work failure.

Organizational interventions are needed to prevent or discontinue counterproductive narcissistic problems in leadership and peer function, especially such problems related to anger, hostility, manipulation, self-expansion, splitting, and control (Book, 2002). For those whose workplaces tend to become the stage for enacting narcissistic self-aggrandizing or self-serving manipulative or hostile strivings, such organizational interventions usually need to precede motivation for therapeutic interventions and personal changes. Some publications have specifically addressed the problems of narcissistic workplace behavior, career pursuits, and leadership strategies (N. W. Brown, 2002; O. Kernberg, 1980, 1998c; Maccoby, 1981).

Work Inhibitions

Unlike those who suffer more obvious self-enhancing, counterproductive, or destructive aspects of work-related narcissistic problems, many people with pathological narcissism struggle with less obvious but usually more painful challenges stemming from shame and self-condemnation of their capabilities and accomplishments. Such work inhibitions can represent an inner inability to pursue a task—even if the task is highly desirable and the person has the ability and competence to perform it. Stage fright and writer's block are examples of such difficulties. Cooper (1998) noted a range of work-related behavior in narcissistic people that contribute to lower performance and inhibitions: chronic or intermittent feelings of boredom and emptiness, and inability to be interested in the work itself and to feel an inner sense of own accomplishments that can lead to sustaining improved experiences of oneself. Work inhibitions can be more overtly expressed in self-defeating and self-sabotaging actions and interpersonal behaviors that obstruct optimal results and accomplishments. The sources of work inhibitions can range from perfectionism and grandiosity to extreme shame and self-criticism. Striving for perfection, in itself a predictor of good accomplishment, can actually encompass an intolerance of imperfection accompanied by tension and fear. It can result in avoidance and passivity, paradoxically experienced as freedom from criticism or imperfection, which may serve to maintain an inner fantasy of perfection (Stark, 1989). While grandiosity and grandiose fantasies for some people are the source of and motivation for accomplishments, for others grandiosity can contribute to feelings of impossibility and unattainability.

Case vignette

Ms. P, a capable and hard-working financial planner in her mid thirties, associated with a progressive investment company, was presented with a peculiar work-related problem. After each accomplishment and step up in her career, something that she had intensely desired and worked hard to reach, she found herself feeling empty and self-critical and unable to enjoy her success. She described a paradoxical experience: on the one hand, she felt that she did not deserve her reward/promotion, and on the other hand, she felt that she had not received enough, that is, that she should have received a higher promotion or a better reward. In other words, Ms. P was unable to maintain an inner feeling of satisfaction and pride in her actual accomplishments. She also admitted that she was hypersensitive to others' comments and evaluations of her performance, envious of others' progress and accomplishments, and constantly worried about being surpassed. Ms. P felt a relentless urge to search for something more, higher, and better. This pattern contributed to disruptions in her professional life and had an impace on Ms. P's private life, as she was constantly looking for better partners. Intensive work in psychotherapy, which focused on anger, shame, and self-criticism, helped Ms. P see a repetitious pattern of trying to please and feeling unable to do so successfully. This pattern, which originated in her relationship to her demanding and distant father, led to underachievement for this intelligent and skilled woman, and it had a damaging impact on her long-term professional growth and development. Gradually being able to contain feelings of self-acceptance, pride, and self-worth and modulate her self-critical attacks, especially related to her body and sexuality, made it possible for Ms. P to begin to enjoy accomplishments, accept praise, and stop the relentless striving for the next promotion. She also cautiously began to pursue more close friendships.

The importance of differentiating between work-related inhibitions due to lack of skills and inhibitions that are related to narcissistic or other personal problems was highlighted in a thought-provoking article on executive coaching. Steven Berglas (2002) made an important distinction between "a problem executive" who can be trained to function effectively and an "executive with a problem" who can best be helped by psychotherapy. Work-inhibiting narcissistic problems can easily be misunderstood as performance problems due to lack the following: assertiveness, a capacity for limit setting and delegation, and interpersonal inefficiency. However, underlying narcissistic problems related to control, intimacy, self-esteem, and anger may be vastly misinterpreted and neglected in the process of coaching, performance enhancing, and assertiveness training. Berglas discussed the negative and sometimes devastating organizational consequences of treating the executives' "symptoms" rather than the underlying problems or disorders.

Case vignette

Mrs. K, a well-educated woman in her mid thirties, had for several years been unable to advance beyond entry-level positions in her professional field of library science. She had on several occasions contacted the director of the human resources department, who suggested some conflict resolution interventions and meetings with her supervisor and a third independent consultant to improve communication and find new avenues for career advancement. However, Mrs. K never found these meetings helpful, and, increasingly dissatisfied with her situation, she sought psychotherapy to further explore the problem in hope of some change. Mrs. K felt underutilized, victimized, and unable to utilize her good education and extensive knowledge, her high professional ambitions, and her capability in project management. As the psychotherapy progressed, Mrs. K expressed more hostility toward several supervisors with whom she had experienced a similar pattern of escalating conflicts. She felt that these supervisors, all female—had less education than she, were controlling, did not like Mrs. K, and were envious of her because of her intelligence and the gains and connections she had made in the workplace.

With further explorations of this pattern, Mrs. K began to describe her relationship to her mother, a possessive, strong-willed, determined woman who had worked hard to put Mrs. K through the best schools. While advancing academically, Mrs. K had increasing conflicts with her mother. She felt guilty for having advanced ahead of her mother who did not have a higher education, and frustrated with what she considered her mother's narrow-mindedness, simple manners, and envy of successful people. She also felt

increasingly ashamed of her background and had problems maintaining an inner continuity of her self and her own progress, feeling as if she did not deserve or was unable to move on in her life.
Apparently this inner conflict was enacted vis-à-vis her supervisors,
causing a self-perpetuating pattern of career traps. While working
through these feelings of disturbed entitlement, shame, and anger,
and on separating this inner conflict from her professional activities
and interactions in the workplace, Mrs. K was able to find a new
position with a career track involving independent grant application
and project management. She felt more in charge of her situation,
improved her collaboration with peers and supervisors, and felt less
angry and trapped.

An inability to hold on to a sense of pride, accomplishment, and competence can disrupt a person's professional performance, self-esteem, and
capacity to collaborate. In a series of articles on stage fright, Glenn Gabbard (1979, 1983, 1997) discussed the narcissistic complexity of accomplishments and especially the role of shame associated with performance.
Stage fright can be related to separation-individuation and "the fear that
asserting oneself as a separate individual will result in withdrawal of love
and admiration by maternal figures, [that is], the audience" (Gabbard,
1979, p. 391). Besides fear of abandonment, Gabbard identified several
sources of performance-related shame and anxiety: the dread of aloneness, fear of exposing forbidden pleasures related to performing, fear of
success, fear of exposure of inadequacy and of being ridiculed, and fears
related to looking and showing (voyeurism and exhibitionism; Gabbard,
1997). In addition, fear of loss of control and fear of autonomy, aggression, destructiveness, and others' envy may contribute to paralyzing, disabling symptoms that disrupt or prevent successful performance (Gabbard, 1983). The following situational vignette illustrates a hidden but
stifling expression of a narcissistic conflict centering on accomplishment,
exhibitionism, and shame accompanied by hostile self-critical attacks.

Case vignette

Mr. P, a 34-year-old unmarried chemical engineer, very intelligent
and devoted but shy and inhibited, had worked for several hours

over the phone with Ms. S, a computer specialist located in a different department in the huge corporate plant. Together they had successfully solved a complex problem in one of the company's computer-generated chemical devices. Mr. P was now walking over to another part of the plant feeling competent, proud, and satisfied with his accomplishment, a combination of affects and experiences of himself that he seldom managed to hold on to as a cohesive experience over sustained period of time. Unexpectedly, he met Mr. M, who said with a big smile: "You can't imagine what Ms. S said about you!" Within a fraction of a second the following sequence of devastating internal experiences occurred in Mr. P: First he thought, " Ahhh, Ms. S likes me, and maybe she would like a date with me." He immediately felt terrified thinking that he would fail and end up being rejected and criticized by Ms. S. Subsequently, a painful feeling of deep shame, failure, and inferiority hit Mr. P, and he began to shake and perspire. In response to Mr. M, he heard himself saying: "Would she like to date me??" This uncontrolled and unintended comment was followed by an increasing feeling of "falling down through the floor," resulting in worsening feelings of shame and inadequacy. As Mr. M in a friendly and encouraging way responded, "You can ask her. She is sitting over there," the cumulative bottom stage was reach for Mr. P: His face was red, his heart pounded, he had difficulties breathing, and he quickly walked back to his desk. He felt stupid, enraged, and deeply ashamed of himself. His colleagues sympathetically asked how he was doing, and Mr. P made a stuttering comment about a sense of inner failure. Mr. P never found out what Ms. S actually had said about him. Further explorations of Mr. P's difficulties revealed not only anxiety related to his sexual performance, but also his fear of rejection and fear of competing with and surpassing male peers out of fear of their envy and retaliation.

Long-term treatment focusing on shame and rage helped Mr. P to be more flexible and comfortable in interpersonal relationships, especially with women. He also pursued a long-term interest in theater and joined an amateur theater group, which gave him ample opportunities to explore and manage his strong feelings and self-experiences when presenting himself in front of other people.

Corrective Experiences

For many people the workplace can offer opportunities for corrective experiences that can adjust unrealistic and unproductive narcissistic strivings into more healthy, productive long-term goals with increased capacity for genuine accomplishments. In a long-term follow-up study of narcissistic patients (Ronningstam, Gunderson, & Lyons, 1995), we found that achievements are the most common corrective life events contributing to improvement in pathological narcissism. Graduations, promotions, recognitions, acceptance to schools, programs, or positions often reduce the need for unrealistic grandiose fantasies and exaggerations of talents and personal qualities. Such events also lead to changes in interpersonal responses such as decreased arrogance and devaluation.

Case vignette

Mr. N, an intelligent, reserved but arrogant 25-year-old man, had suffered from depression for several years. Although an unusually competent student, he constantly felt unappreciated. He described himself as superior, with feelings of disdain and confusion toward people whose values and standards were different from his own. He also described himself as intellectually unique, stressing his specific theoretical and philosophical perspective and high academic standards. He liked to give teachers and professors a hard time by asking "impossible" questions. He had close friends among his male peers but felt shy and insecure in relating to young women.

Mr. N came from a competitive and successful family background. His father, with whom he had a complicated relationship, was a successful lawyer. He both admired and idealized his father, felt deeply misunderstood by him, and despised him for his demands, values, and expectations. While he envied his father and fantasized about becoming as successful as him, he also felt inferior and took every opportunity to protest against him. After graduate school, Mr. N decided to work as a pizza deliverer, a decision that he considered in line with his "unique life approach." Three years later Mr. N reported several important developments. Individual psychotherapy for 1-1/2 years had focused specifically on insecurity and depression. A new job as a teacher at a community college contributed to important changes in his behavior and attitudes toward himself and others. He had developed techniques for teaching, and he had learned to interact with people and appreciate others' different ideas and values. He also described himself as more tolerant of criticism. His sense of pride reflected more realistic self-appraisals and diminished arrogance. The relationship with his father remained conflicted, but a sincere desire to identify with his competent and successful father had also surfaced. Relations with women had improved, and his girlfriend of 2 years had greatly contributed to improving his self-esteem. As Mr. N's experiences of realistic competence and independent, goal-oriented, professional responsibility increased, his narcissistic self-inflation and antagonizing and devaluating behavior toward others decreased, and his capacity for mutual interpersonal relations could develop.

We also found that corrective disillusionment may involve work-related changes and contribute to a more realistic self-appraisal and professional goals. Corrective disillusionments involve experiences that are incompatible with and challenge the previous grandiose self-experience, bringing the view of self into greater congruence with actual talents, abilities, and status. Such experiences may reflect the realization of personal, intellectual, or vocational limitations, failure to achieve life goals or conform to narcissistically determined ideals and standards, or even personal losses or lost opportunities in life. However, the impact of such experiences must not be too adverse. If especially severe and experienced without support, narcissistic pathologies may actually worsen.

Case vignette

Mr. O, an executive in his mid forties, considered himself to be goal-oriented and superintelligent, with strong, Puritan values, quick reasoning skill, and extraordinary leadership capacity. Although happily married with two teenage sons and a younger daughter, he viewed himself as a loner, not interested in wasting time with meaningless social activities. As a top manager in a small company, he was boastful, self-praising, and self-centered. He consistently devalued the social acumen of others but did admit that he envied their social belonging. When his company suddenly underwent a major expansion, Mr. O was sent to a very challenging business school for continuing education to meet the company's new needs. Used to being the most intellectually accomplished person in any group, Mr. O was stunned at discovering the exceptionally high intellectual level among the other graduate students. With humility, admiration, and some envy, he accepted his own B+ grades. At follow-up, Mr. O was in the process of returning to a new position in his company. He described feeling remarkably more humble, with less intense aggressive, bragging, and self-inflating behavior. In his own appraisal, he had reached the maximum of his personal and professional capacity. Satisfied with his results in graduate school and feeling strongly motivated to take on new professional tasks in his company, he noticed a new sense of vulnerability and less of his usual courage. Facing personal and professional limitations was enormously challenging for Mr. O's self-esteem. With the sustained support of his loyal wife, and his own personal flexibility and capacity to integrate initially unacceptable aspects of himself, he was able to bring a grandiose self-image more in line with reality.

Career Interruptions—A Narcissistic Humiliation

Professional people who become psychiatrically ill often find themselves unable to meet their previous high standard of vocational performance and achievement. Their experience can be described as an interrupted career, that is, a temporary or permanent inability to participate professionally in regular vocational tasks and contexts. Job loss and unemployment have usually been associated with layoffs due to economic fluctuations, company restructuring, or other factors less related to individual competence. The psychosocial impact of job loss may involve such narcissistic challenges as undermining of self-esteem, change or loss of support network, and uncovering of preexisting problems or deficits, including psychiatric disorders that were compensated for or counterbalanced through work (Kates, Greiff, & Hagen, 1990). Studies have found that personality structure, that is, mood of interaction (Viinamaeki, Niskanen, & Koskela, 1995), and personality coping style, such as affectivity and avoidance, predict the individual's capacity to handle occupational stress and to remain mentally healthy during the experience of unemployment (Roskies, Louis-Guerin, & Fournier, 1993; Smari, Arason, Hafsteinsson, & Ingimarsson, 1997). No studies have yet focused on career interruption or job loss occurring as a consequence of the onset of a psychiatric disorder and accompanying changes in work performance.

Given the importance of work for healthy narcissistic functioning, it is reasonable to assume that a decline in or loss of work role or capacity can lead to a disruption in normal self-esteem regulation and self-cohesiveness. Increased pathological narcissism, such as defensive grandiosity and intense reactions including shame, rage, humiliation, envy, and feelings of inferiority may result. This assumption is further endorsed by clinical observations that intense shame reactions can lead to self-disintegration and depression (Broucek, 1982; Morrison, 1983). In some cases, a job loss can even be experienced as a narcissistic trauma (Simon, 2001), that is, a personal attack or an insult, or an act of deliberate deceitfulness that can evoke rage and revengefulness.

The Interrupted Career Group

The Interrupted Career Group (ICG; Ronningstam & Anick, 2001) was developed as a psychotherapy group for people who had experienced interruptions in their professional activities due to personality disorders and/or affective disorders. We believed that narcissistic reactions to interruption of career and life due to psychiatric illness can have a paralyzing and/or disabling effect. As mentioned above, such reactions include shame, humiliation, rage, envy, and feelings of inferiority. It is plausible that these reactions in themselves, independently or in the presence of a major psychiatric disorder, can prevent the individual from reaching optimal vocational and personal functioning. The ICG was an attempt to treat these emotional obstacles to recovery by using focused group psychotherapy.

The purpose of the ICG was to discuss the emotional and practical difficulties related to resuming personal and vocational activities after a career interruption. However, as people with interrupted careers also were struggling with problems related to low motivation and self-esteem, feelings of failure and severe humiliation and lack of direction in professional and personal life, they usually had difficulties finding adequate treatment modalities. The ICG was specifically designed to fill this niche for professionally experienced and well-educated people whose major psychiatric disorder was relatively stable and well treated. The choice of addressing characterologically related problems in group therapy was supported by reports on treatment of character pathology and shame in this treatment modality (Alonso & Rutan, 1988, 1993). In addition, the use of group approaches as part of a multimodal treatment strategy of personality disorders has proved increasingly valuable (Smith, Ruiz Sancho, & Gunderson, 2000).

All group members had had a period of normal work experience, various levels of achievement or success, and an identity that included a sense of themselves as engaged and successful in a career. People were not enrolled while in psychiatric crisis, and members were expected, during a screening interview, to demonstrate capacities for affect processing. In the screening, members were asked to describe their interruption and to specify an "agenda" and some short-term or long-term goals. The goal could be career resumption, but it could also involve pursuing education, volunteer work, a hobby, or social change depending upon the individual circumstances.

The ICG participants were asked to define their interruption, that is, describe their life and work before the interruption, the events and factors leading up to the interruption, and the consequences and changes caused by the interruption. The participants were also asked to define an agenda, that is, some specific ideas and goals related to what they want to change or pursue in their vocational and personal life. Each group member was asked to define and pursue an integrated track with vocational and/or personal activities that integrated "there and then" with "here and now." In other words, the members were encouraged to discuss what they did and had before, compared with what they are and have now in terms of limitations and losses, interests and experiences, and skills and possibilities, specifically in the context of pursuing a new integrated track. The participants were specifically encouraged to attend to the feelings related to or triggered directly by these pursuits.

The people attending the group addressed specific difficulties in their recovery and reorientation after having experienced an interrupted career due to psychiatric illness. Many of the members had been unemployed or underemployed for several years. Most exhibited a type of distortion that was specific to workplace relationships or opportunities. Approach avoidance to working had become reinforced. This was usually through a cycle of depression leading to failure or loss of motivation, followed by low self-esteem and, in some cases, contributing to increasing withdrawal into passivity and isolation. Further exploration of the nature and content of the members' depression showed that although part of the depression was manageable via a psychopharmacological treatment modality, for most members a major aspect of the depression related to unresolved feelings about the career interruption. These feelings included emptiness, inadequacy, humiliation, rage, shame, envy, and worthlessness. Additional aspects of depression related to unresolved grief over the major losses that followed the interruption, that is, loss of spouse and/or family, social connectedness, and professional creativity. For some members, unresolved conflicts vis-à-vis former employers contributed to severe rumination, revengeful feelings, and difficulties in pursuing new vocational steps. These aspects of the depression seem to cause long-term, inflexible, and maladaptive patterns of inner experiences and behavior that led to additional functional impairment in these otherwise gifted and capable people.

The Group Process   The major therapeutic focus was on the group members' feelings and fluctuations in self-esteem as they related to their efforts in pursuing new steps toward an integrated vocational and personal track. However, people also experienced considerable practical obstacles that obstructed their ability to start up new activities. Consequently, the topics discussed in the group covered a broad range of problems from how to present themselves in an interview with a potential employer to how to manage excessive feelings of inferiority and envy when meeting old classmates at a high school reunion. For those who resumed professional activities, major problems were connected to issues related to their own performance or self-appraisal, explaining time out of work, and interpersonal relations to peers, supervisors, and bosses. For others, self-loathing, contempt, self-criticism, and insecurity or fear of trying new things were prominent. Throughout the group process, members learned how the extensive consequences of interrupted careers could affect most areas of life, including attending children's graduations or weddings, getting through major holidays, or sustaining interest in former leisure activities or hobbies. As members progressed toward their new goals, they usually experienced increased and sometimes overwhelming sadness and grief at what had been lost. Paradoxically, regaining skills and confidence and resuming professional activities in some form led to comparisons of "there and then" with "here and now." Reactions including rage and experiences of unfairness, unacceptability, and discouragement were not uncommon. Intense narcissistic reactiveness—especially shame and anger—to the career interruption was notable in most of the participants. In addition, group members' progress usually involved a substantial period of working through their feelings and experiences related to pathological narcissism, such as defensive superiority, entitlement, enraged revengefulness, and inferiority.

The experience of career interruption provided a point of homogeneity and bonding among the group members, who often commented on the value of discussing the specific problems related to having both an interrupted career and a psychiatric disability with people in a similar situation. They felt understood, supported, and less inhibited by shame and guardedness. Within this experience, however, was considerable diversity based on the duration of the disability, the nature and severity of the psychiatric illness, the degree of achievement attained before the interruption, the patients' character structures and coping methods, and the presence or absence of financial and/or emotional support from family, friends, and employers both before and after the interruption.

Career after Career Interruption

The following case vignettes serve to illustrate the work and progress of group members.

Case vignettes

Mrs. A had lost her own business as an art dealer due to sudden exasperating depression that also uncovered personality problems related to passive submissiveness and inhibited ability to identify and express feelings, especially anger. The professional interruption was accompanied by a divorce. When Mrs. A joined the group, she was isolated and detached from her usual professional, social, and family context and temporarily employed in a small gasoline station and auto mechanic shop, a totally unrelated vocational activity far below her previous level of income and functioning. However, Mrs. A had a survival instinct and did actually feel a certain enjoyment and pride in managing what she described as an odd type of work in a typical male environment. The experience of increasing technical competence in this unrelated field actually seemed to help Mrs. A ward off the suicidal feelings she had struggled with since her divorce. While in the group she made failed attempts to get back into positions with some connection to her previous business world.

She continued to work actively on her feelings of humiliation, rage, shame, and powerlessness related to the major interruption in her over 20-year-long career and the loss of her marriage. After 14 months of active participation in the group, she was able to find employment in a progressive company where she could use her interactional and business skills while working in a more structured and less competitive environment.

Mr. B was in his late forties when his career as a social worker was drastically interrupted and his whole life situation markedly and quickly changed due to bipolar disorder. However, despite illness, he had been able to hold on to low-pay temporary positions that somewhat related to his previous profession. Having lost contact with his four sons, who refused to meet with him after he got ill, and learning that his wife, who divorced him, had remarried, Mr. B felt deeply humiliated, empty, and lost. He spent a lot of free time in bed dozing or sleeping. During thorough and long-term work in the group, Mr. B reconnected with his sons, began dating and meeting new people, and took recertification courses to enable him to reapply for licensure as a social worker. As his life progressed, Mr. B became aware of how each step toward an active and integrated personal life and return to his professional life was accompanied by confrontations with past experiences, consequences of the interruption, and realizations of the substantial losses he had experienced. For each step, Mr. B systematically discussed his overwhelming feelings of grief, humiliation, shame, envy, and inferiority. After a year and a half of ICG therapy Mr. B terminated the group, entered a permanent full-time position in his former professional field, and moved out of a house for the disabled into his own apartment.

Ms. C, an ambitious, hardworking, 45-year-old owner of a fashion store had decided to sell her business after having suffered from several episodes of depression during which she had put her business on hold. Ms. C, who was normally a matter-of-fact, outgoing, and cheerful person who enjoyed her business and customers immensely, was initially open to a major reorientation in her life. However, as she gradually realized that the option of selling her business felt like a huge loss and failure, she began to explore other alternatives: pursuing co-ownership, selling the business and staying as an employee, or looking for other types of work. Ms. C worked intensively in the group on her feelings of inferiority and deep sense of loss of a stimulating and rewarding environment. After a few weeks she decided to reopen her business part-time and pursue a well-structured and balanced work schedule adjusted to her mood disorder and her need to prevent exasperation due to overwork.

Mr. D was a 40-year-old conscientious and successful financial consultant, who over a period of a couple of years developed a barely noticeable bipolar disorder with slightly elevated mood. With hindsight, Mr. D realized that he had reacted by getting overly involved in work and in certain clients. He made a serious professional mistake and had to close his business. Mr. D was a very down-to-earth and matter-of-fact man who had a broad experience of different types of labor and working environments before entering a professional career. He also had an unusual capacity for personal independence, adjustment, and tolerance of humiliation. Nevertheless, Mr. D's experience of shame and personal loss was overwhelming. The father of a 5-year-old son with a very supportive wife, he decided to devote his time to parenting his son, while he readjusted to his psychological and financial limitations and explored possible new avenues. After a year of intensive work in the ICG and other therapy modalities, he decided to pursue a graduate degree in computer science, a track he chose specifically because it involved less stressful interactions and the possibilities of independent and more structured work.

Mr. E, a man in his mid thirties, had just become the vice director of a financial investment company when he began having severely incapacitating depressive episodes. This was accompanied by memory impairment and exasperating personality disorder symptoms. He also began having chronic suicidal ideations and, after a serious suicide attempt, he was forced to give up his profession indefinitely. Although married to a supportive wife and living in an active neighborhood where he could do volunteer tasks on his own, Mr. E found himself at a total professional and personal loss. Since his early teens, he had relied on his considerable capacity for working and had overcome personal difficulties and gained self-esteem and self-respect due to his major achievements. In this new situation as a disabled person, he struggled with overwhelming feelings of shame, self-hatred, worthlessness, inferiority, and enraged cynicism. Every attempt to do alternative paid work was accompanied by intense rage and self-criticism. Long-term work (18 months) in the group with specific focus on self-hatred, shame, envy, and inferiority made it possible for Mr. E to gain some self-acceptance and begin to do structured and well-defined tasks within his profession on a volunteer basis for a friend's business.

Mrs. F was a woman in her late forties who, despite several years of struggle with a mood disorder, had managed to develop a significant career as a researcher and project manager within the biochemical industry. The divorced mother of two adult children, she was considered to be a friendly, sociable, and easy-going person with many friends and she had good relationships with her ex-husband and family. However, while experiencing increasing problems in a relationship to a man she expected to marry, she began to have brief episodes of severe depression, excessive self-doubt, and inability to attend to work. She also began to leave work or stay home from work without prior announcement. This pattern was accompanied by extreme and severely incapacitating feelings of guilt and remorse vis-à-vis her managers and the program director and fear of losing her job when she returned. This pattern worsened and led to her losing three high positions in different companies within a short period of time. When starting the group, Mrs. F was working with a package delivery service while applying for numerous jobs in her professional field all over the country. Mrs. F engaged in long-term work on accepting and understanding the interruption in her professional career. She also discussed the grief related to the gradual realization of the loss of her career, and the shame related to her new vocational track in delivery service, which, she admitted with considerable embarrassment, she actually had started to like. The work contributed to both financial and personal stability, she had begun to make some friends and was highly appreciated among peers and supervisors.

Change and Cure Through the ICG

It seemed that a major curative factor was related to the specific composition of the group, that is, people who had experienced a career or a sustained period of healthy high functioning that was interrupted. The members easily identified with each other and shared experiences and problems.

The group stimulated a cognitive and affective tension between "there and then" and "here and now" within and between members of the group. This particular tension rekindled memories of experiences and feelings from the past (i.e., "I used to do/have/like this . . .") that seemed to reactivate the participants' motivation and mental energy while providing a perspective and understanding of individual efforts and difficulties that helped diminish self-criticism. In addition, the combination of mutual understanding and supportive interactions among the members and the tension created between them as each one reported progressive steps also seemed to reactivate their motivation. Other helpful interactions included the feedback on how other group members saw their strengths and weaknesses, and the fact that members who succeeded in reaching their goals or getting a job served as role models for others. Obviously, this motivation, combined with the emotionally open and supportive atmosphere, was necessary for enabling the members to begin to take steps toward emotional integration and vocationally related change. However, for some members whose affect regulation was too impaired and/or whose illness was less stable or well managed, this motivation did not occur or became too overwhelming.

A few participants for whom the interruption had occurred recently, or whose attitude to the interruption was less influenced by shame and humiliation, were able to utilize the group in a effective way to find resolutions to their interruption within a relatively short time. However, most group members required several months to fully benefit from the group process, implement desired changes, or work through intensive feelings related to their interruption.

The participants' progressive work and development over a 2.5-year period were evident. Two-thirds of the participants used the group to discuss feelings and efforts connected to resuming an integrated track that resulted in actual changes. These changes were notable either in vocational/educational/volunteer activities and emotional functioning, or mainly in emotional functioning and less in vocational/educational/

volunteer activities. The people who did not find the group beneficial in promoting change in any of these areas were too ill, had acute relapses, or were unable or unmotivated to pursue the group. However, several of these members still actively participated in and contributed to the group process and the other members' work in a constructive and supportive way.

As the ICG has progressed, it has been considered an important component in a multimodal aftercare program for people who are facing major changes or interruption in their vocational/professional activities due to a psychiatric disorder.

Conclusions

As much as narcissistic investment in work is a crucial part of healthy individual functioning and exceptional accomplishments, it can also develop into the opposite, that is, counterproductive working behavior, destructive leadership, and stifling inhibitions. The purpose of this chapter was to discuss how to identify pathological narcissism and narcissistic reactions in the context of vocational/professional functioning and interactions in workplace. In addition, career interruptions can evoke strong feelings of shame, envy, rage, inferiority, and humiliation that in and of themselves undermine the capacity and motivation for resuming work activities. An interactive group process focusing specifically on such feelings related to experiences of the interrupted career can contribute to improve emotional and vocational functioning.

7

My Way or No Way!

Narcissism and Suicide

Although the risk of suicide attempt and completed suicide usually has been associated with mood and substance-abuse disorders, the proportion of deaths among people with personality disorders has actually been estimated to be between 5% and 10% (Black, Warrack, & Winkur, 1985; Miles 1977). A recent psychological autopsy study of suicide in 15–24-year-olds in the United Kingdom found that nearly 30% had personality disorders and 55% had traits of personality disorders (Houston, Hawton, & Shepperd, 2001). Four other European studies confirmed that the presence of personality disorders is both an important risk factor for chronic suicidality with repeated suicide attempts and a predictor for suicide reattempts (5 years) and completed suicides (Cording & Huebner Liebermann, 2000; Hansen, Wang, Stage, & Kragh-Sorensen, 2003; Johnsson-Fridell, Öjehagen, & Träskman-Bendz, 1996; Schmidtke et al., 2000). While suicidal and parasuicidal behavior have foremost been associated with borderline personality disorder (*DSM-IV*; Gunderson & Ridolfi, 2001), the antisocial personality disorder is considered to have the highest suicide rate (10–15%; Dahl, 1998).

With regard to NPD, there is clinical agreement that narcissistic patients are prone to suicidal behavior. C. J. Perry (1990) noted that "the extreme vulnerability to loss of self-esteem coupled with dysphoria in response to failure, criticism and humiliation should put these individuals at high risk for suicide attempts" (p. 159). One study (Apter et al., 1993) found that as many as 23.3% of young males who committed suicide had a diagnosis of NPD. Other follow-up studies (McGlashan & Heinssen, 1989; Stone, 1989) have found that co-occurrence of narcissistic features or NPD increased the risk for suicide in borderline patients. Compared to borderline patients (Gunderson & Ridolfi, 2001), people with NPD are rarely overtly self-destructive, and they have significantly lower levels of suicidal ideation (Morey & Jones, 1998; Plakun, 1989). Furthermore, parasuicidal behavior and suicidal threats are not characteristic of NPD. Narcissistic people do not usually act to elicit others' attention or with intentions to manipulate others. A major difference between the two types of personality disorders is noticeable in the relationship to the therapist. While the borderline patient pulls the therapist right into the core of the action of suicide, the narcissistic patient tends to keep suicidality as a protective shield vis-à-vis the therapist. For the narcissistic patient, suicidality serves as an inner regulator, that is, to compensate for loss of self-esteem and impaired affect regulation—intolerance or impaired capacity to process affects, especially feelings of rage, shame, and inferiority. Suicidal ideations may be hidden and effectively sealed over a long time. They may also be embedded in chronic severe feelings of shame; that is, originally there was a shaming experience triggering the initial feelings or act of suicidality that may or may not be fully conscious and known.

Studies of the relationship between narcissism and suicide have suggested two major avenues. Henseler (1974, 1981; see also Etzersdorfer, 2001) highlighted the role of narcissistic vulnerability and fragile self-esteem regulation and considered the function of suicide as an act to save the self-feeling or self-regard. O. Kernberg (1984) and Kohut (1972) added the role of self-directed aggression, suggesting that narcissistic rage attacks can arise from humiliating or threatening experiences or other injuries to the self. O. Kernberg (1992) also noted that ego-syntonic suicidal tendencies can emerge "with the underlying (conscious or unconscious) fantasy that to be able to take one's life reflects superiority and a triumph over the usual fear of pain and death" (p. 78). In severe forms of NPD, with malignant narcissism (O. Kernberg, 1984, 1992), the patient's chronic suicidal preoccupation may be accompanied by cold, sadistic, vengeful satisfaction and a secret or overt triumph and superiority over the clinician, a way to execute power and control. Such patients can have increased suicidality when they feel that the therapist has been specifically helpful (negative therapeutic reaction; O. Kernberg, 2001), because those experiences may evoke feelings of shame caused by anticipated dependency, and envy of the therapist's capacity to be helpful. This can become an invisible nightmare for the clinician.

This chapter provides an overview of the specific dynamics of suicidal ideations and behavior in narcissistic patients. Diagnostic guidelines for identifying and exploring narcissistic aspects of their suicidal ideations are discussed, as well as some specifically challenging diagnostic and treatment considerations.

The Narcissistic Meaning of Suicide

People who commit suicide have usually been considered to be depressed and unhappy, or to feel deep hopelessness and guilt, or to be seriously mentally ill. However, in narcissistic patients suicidal ideations and behavior can often be less related or even entirely unrelated to depression (O. Kernberg, 1992; Maltsberger, 1998). Because of the particular structural deformities in narcissistic disorders—the presence of a pathological grandiose self with accompanying narcissistic vulnerability, and self-esteem regulation specifically geared toward protection of the grandiose self-image—suicidal behavior in narcissistic patients can have several specific dynamic meanings. (1) The fantasy of suicide can raise the self-esteem because it supports an illusion of mastery and control ("I fear nothing, not even death"). (2) Suicidal behavior can shield against anticipated narcissistic threats and injuries ("death before dishonor"). (3) Suicidal impulses may stem from aggressive, revengeful, and controlling attitudes or impulses, that is, "my way or no way" or "I'll show you." (4) They can also arise from a grandiose delusion of indestructibility. (5) Further, they can express the wish to attack or destroy an imperfect, failing, intolerable self. These attitudes can occur in combination, for example, " I destroy my failing body so that my perfect soul can survive" or "by killing myself before the disgrace I can remain perfect and in control" (Ronningstam & Maltsberger, 1998, p. 262). In addition, the idea of suicide can represent an illusion of turning passive humiliation into active mastery (Rothstein, 1980), or superiority and a triumph over the usual fear of pain and death (O. Kernberg, 1992), or a fantasy of becoming "one with death" in which an idealized omnipotent internal object has a desire to destroy the self (Rush, 2000). The transference of these patients often reflects an identification with primitive sadistic object representations, that is, internalized negative and punitive early experiences of others, which are enacted for purposes of revenge and control. Self-destructive and suicidal activities can provide means of asserting power and triumph over the therapist (O. Kernberg, 1984).

Maltsberger (1998) highlighted the role of unstable self-representations that can contribute to a split between the body and other representations, leading to a "not-me" sense or objectification of the body with an unusual risk of physical, aggressive attacks with a suicidal outcome. He also noted that self-dysregulation, that is, dysfunctional regulation of self-criticism, affects, self-esteem, and so forth, can lead to inner self-attacks that can have suicidal consequences. Based on M. Klein's (1958) formulations, Maltsberger (1998) described two types of suicide with relevance to narcissistic disorders. The first is the metamorphic suicide based on the fantasy of suicide as an act of transformation from an intolerable present into a better future. This suicide can occur "in patients whose grandiosity, cruelty, and object detachment rise to malignant proportions" (p. 336). It reflects the realistic perception of the incoherent self as changing. In the second type, the execution suicide, a fantasy is enacted in which the unaccepted or intolerable body is attacked by a superior and extremely harsh executive superego to free the good world from such badness (pp. 339–340).

Suicidal Behavior in the Absence of Depression

Although suicidality usually has been associated with depressed mood, the connection between suicidality and depression in narcissistic patients may not be easily noticeable or even present. In other words, the usual clinical definition of depression that requires the presence of several typical features is not readily applicable. Depressed mood (feelings of sadness, hopelessness, etc.), loss of interest and pleasure, loss of appetite, sleep disturbances, psychomotor changes, decreased energy and fatigue, impaired concentration, and feelings of worthlessness and guilt may not be noticeable or overtly present in the suicidal narcissistic individual. The difficulties assessing depression in the presence of narcissistic pathology are mainly caused by these patients' tendencies to hide and deny such symptoms. Grandiosity, feelings of shame, and interpersonal conflicts can help to effectively seal underlying feelings of worthlessness or hopelessness or other signs of depression. In addition, the specific narcissistic dynamics and functions of suicide, especially when involving rage and revenge, may also in certain cases preclude symptoms of depression. All these circumstances may cause the clinician to disregard possible signs of suicidality.

Recent studies have given further hints on how chronic suicidality can occur without the presence of depression (Bronish, 1996; O. Kernberg, 1993b; Maltsberger, 1998;). They have suggested that people can feel suicidal and even kill themselves, not in an effort to escape intolerable feelings related to severe acute depression, that is, hopelessness, despair, pain, or anguish, but because of an underlying sense of superiority or feelings of rage, or because of other personal reasons for acting in a destructive or self-destructive way. Some of these people may be very high functioning with a good sense of identity and good reality testing.

In a study of three young men with narcissistic disorders who made near-lethal suicide attempts without conscious intent to kill themselves and without manifestations or experience of depression (Ronningstam & Maltsberger, 1998), a combination of characteristics and circumstances were identified that can contribute to high suicide risk in narcissistic patients. Each patient was admitted to an inpatient unit and underwent suicide risk consultation, diagnostic evaluation, and brief psychotherapy.

Case vignettes

Mr. A, a 29-year-old law student, spitefully tried to hang himself during a visit in his paramour's home while she was on the telephone with her new fiancée. Leaving a suicide note where he believed she would quickly find it, he went into her kitchen, attached a rope to a closet door, and hanged himself. He wrongly assumed she would rush in to rescue him within minutes. Fifteen to twenty minutes passed, however, before the girlfriend discovered him, by which time he was severely anoxic. Mr. A later described having been distressed, confused, and angry for several months, ever since she had announced her plans to marry another man. She had continued to see Mr. A, maintained a sexual relationship with him, told him to keep their intimacy secret, and had given him ambiguous and sometimes promising messages. After the hanging, Mr. A unwaveringly denied he ever had any intention to kill himself. He further denied ever weighing the terrible risk of his decision to stage a "mock" hanging. He had been convinced he would hang in his rope only a couple of minutes. On admission to the hospital he steadfastly denied having had symptoms of depression in recent months. He said the prime purpose of the hanging was to make a statement to his former girlfriend, to "scare her or shake her up," maybe to make her change her decision regarding future marriage. He had also felt a strong wish to be rescued by her. Mr. A's father had made numerous suicide attempts in the past, and Mr. A had actually rescued him twice.

Mr. B, a 22-year-old recent college graduate with a complex psychiatric history (including several hospitalizations and suicidal gestures in reaction to stressful situations in the past), claimed that a self-hanging that nearly killed him was actually part of a film project and not a suicide attempt at all. He had decided to film himself with a video camera, he said, while faking a suicide attempt. He had intended to get the film exhibited on a national television show. He threw a rope over a ceiling-beam and placed a chair underneath, set a video camera going in front of him, and put a noose around his neck. He vigorously flexed his neck muscles to simulate death agony. The chair "slipped," the rope broke, and Mr. B fell to the ground, unconscious. Discovered by relatives, Mr. B vehemently denied any suicidal intent. He was surprised and annoyed at the response of others to what he considered to be his movie project. He later admitted to curiosity about the meaning of life and death and said he wanted to explore the intermediate state between the two. At the time of his hanging, Mr. B faced a number of separations and losses: His psychotherapist had begun to terminate with him, he himself had decided to terminate group therapy, several of his close friends were in the process of moving to other parts of the country, and he had just attended a relative's funeral. Nonetheless, he denied that these events had any relationship whatever to his hanging.

Mr. C, a 22-year-old extraordinarily intelligent microbiology graduate student, swallowed between one and two milligrams of potassium cyanide that he had taken from a chemistry laboratory. After a moment he vomited and went to sleep, wakening the following morning in time for an appointment with his visiting mother. Mr. C denied that anything had upset him that might have triggered his lethal behavior, but much later acknowledged that the visit from his mother was remarkably coincidental in the timing of his cyanide ingestion. He denied having had symptoms of depression beforehand, and there were no signs of psychosis or delusions. Thoughts of death and the meaning of life had preoccupied him for several years. For some time he had toyed with the idea of suicide to discover whether there was an afterlife, but dispassionately, more or less as a research project. He terminated a relationship with a girlfriend because he felt it interfered with his suicide experiment. Paradoxically, he denied having wishes or intentions to end his life, and he stated that he was making a scientific test about the nature of life after death. Afterward, he said his experience of being so close to death actually strengthened his wish to live. In discussing his lethal behavior, Mr. C consistently remained emotionally detached and without visible feeling. High expectations from his father, who had in the past expressed a similar interest in suicide and who considered suicide attempts a normal aspect of philosophical curiosity, had driven Mr. C's exceptionally intensive and successful academic career. Mr. C's mother was a disturbed person: Deluded and depressed, she was subject to very aggressive moods and constantly tried to manipulate and control family members. The mother's illness had contributed to the parents' marital estrangement. Mr. C. unrealistically felt responsible for this and had been trying, unsuccessfully, to mediate between his parents.

Common Characteristics

These young men consistently denied primary suicidal intent. Each rationalized his suicidal behavior: one said it was a hostile prank, another claimed he was staging a movie performance, and the third declared he was making a scientific experiment. All of them denied having felt depressed at the time of their bizarre behavior, before or afterward. None met the diagnostic criteria for major depression, and none showed any major clinical manifestations of depression during the evaluations. Failure to acknowledge the high risk of bodily injury and death in connection to lethal behavior was striking in all three patients, who minimized, rationalized, or even denied both cognitive and emotional signals indicating risk of injury or loss of life. There were obvious interpersonal stressors present (loss of fiancée, loss of several friends and roommates in the context of terminating treatment, and unrealistic responsibility for parents) that appeared to drive the self-attacks in each case but that were dismissed or minimized by each patient. In addition, these young men also had extremely unrealistic attitudes toward death and dying.

Narcissistic Features

There are some notable features of pathological narcissism in these three patients. First, they all seemed to fail in the normal narcissistic self-preserving and self-protecting functions, showing an incapacity to protect the body or to acknowledge deadly risk. This is consistent with body indifference and alienation, but less obviously suggestive of bodily self-hate. Second, they were all incapable of identifying and responding adaptively to painful life events, that is, experiences that challenge the narcissistic person's self-experience and character defense and interfere with narcissistic strivings or a sense of specialness, capability, or importance. Several common features of narcissistic psychopathology may contribute to this state of affairs: the narcissistic patient's (a) impaired capacity for empathy, that is, failure to grasp the emotional meaning of the *inner psychological state* and experiences of other people as well as an inability to tolerate and separate oneself from ones own feelings (see chapters 2 and 4 this volume); (b) intense rage reactions in response to defeats; and the usually more hidden characterological vulnerability distinguished by (c) hypersensitivity to others' reactions, (d) deep feelings of inferiority, and (e) sensitivity to loss and rejection. Each of these suicide-related acts seemed to a greater or lesser degree to reflect (f) a grandiose fantasy and a narcissistic pursuit. Each patient was intent on influencing the uninfluenceable, exploring the unexplorable, or creating the uncreatable. Each act can be understood as a magical effort to overcome unsurpassable interpersonal obstacles and to reach impossible goals. In addition, each patient believed and acted as if he was immortal.

Facets of the Suicidal Narcissistic Patient

Impaired Affect Regulation

Why can suicidal behavior in narcissistic patients take place especially in the absence of depression? One explanation can be found in the impaired affect regulation associated with narcissistic pathology (see also chapter

4 this volume). Krystal (1998) describes pathological narcissistic compensatory processes arising from such impaired regulatory functions. He
writes of "processes that promote denial of failures, isolation or a splitting
off of intolerable affects or somatic symptoms, maintenance of omnipotent or grandiose fantasies, and experiences of superiority or belief in
invulnerability" (p. 307). Schore (1994) referred to the failure in persons
with narcissistic disorders to develop adequate affect regulation with the
help of self-objects. Such patients lack an essential unconscious, psychobiological capacity to stabilize the self-structure against stressful levels
of stimulation and affect arousal. Normal persons with adequate regulatory structure are able to "neutralize grandiosity, regulate excitement, or
modulate narcissistic distress" (p. 427). In the absence of such structure,
negative affects such as rage and shame can not be tolerated or regulated,
and damaged relationships with others prove difficult to reestablish and
repair. Clearly, this specific combination of narcissistic and affect pathology can underpin sudden self-inflicted death in the absence of depression.
Fonagy (1993) explored the defensive function of aggression in protecting
identity and the reflective self. He suggested that aggression and destructiveness in patients with severe borderline and narcissistic disorders
have lost their protective function and become linked to self-expression.
The capacity for meta-cognitive control, reflective self-functioning, and
mentalization that can help protect against narcissistic injury (Fonagy,
1999, pp. 57–58) has not developed in suicidal narcissistic patients. The
person is unable to think and reflect beyond the immediate experience
and unable to use aggression as a protective shield against overwhelming
experiences, thoughts, and feelings. Furthermore, aggression becomes the
major mode of self-expression activated in a variety of situations, and the
person's capacity to reflect and understand the consequences of aggressive and self-destructive actions is impaired. Fonagy (1993) noted that a
boy's self-sabotaging behavior could be deadly; "his primitive reflective
self did not see the death of his body as leading to the death of his mental
self" (p. 481).

Dissociation

Why at a certain point can grandiose fantasies be acted upon in a deadly
manner? The mental states into which some narcissistic patients can
enter are probably dissociation. One group of mental processes (those
driving the suicidal behavior and the associated affects) can be split off

from the rest of the personality. In addition, certain operations of the ego, for example, cognitive functioning (judgment) and reality testing, appear to have been shut down or sequestered. Dissociative phenomena in suicide have now begun to attract more attention (Orbach, Lotem-Peleg, & Kedem, 1995), while previous reports discuss such states in terms of objectification of the body image followed by a depressive attack upon an enemy (Maltsberger, 1993). Patients with narcissistic features, such as the three presented above, can apparently reach a state where they do not seem concerned that their self-attacks can destroy their body. Instead, they become oblivious to any bodily danger because they do not experience themselves as suicidal at all, or else believe they are immortal. In these patients, the dissociative state led to a situation in which the grandiose suicidal intentions were acted upon, and whatever reality and self-protective functions prevented suicidal actions earlier were disconnected. In other words, by the process of dissociation these patients could remain grandiose in their intent, deny danger, and act upon their suicidal ideations in a life-threatening dangerous manner.

Shame and Rage

Why can a dissociative state accompanied by suicidal behavior arise in a patient with a narcissistic personality disorder who usually has high and intact ego strength and cognitive functioning? Recent research on the role and effect of primitive shame and rage in narcissistic disorders, that is, shame and rage that are less differentiated and originating from an infantile developmental phase, suggests an answer (Broucek, 1982; Kohut, 1972, pp. 394–396; Kohut, 1977, p. 77; Schore, 1991). Moreover, the role of shame in suicide has been reported in both suicide studies and psychoanalytic studies. One study (Lester, 1998) found that shame was more strongly associated with suicidality than was guilt, especially among men; in another study by Hassan (1995; see Hastings, Northman, & Tangney, 2000), shame and guilt, defined as a sense of disgrace from failure to meet obligations or social expectations, was a precipitating trigger in 7% of completed suicides. In addition, feelings of shame were probably also involved in the most common cause of suicide in this study: "a sense of failure in life." Lansky (1991) related shame to the loss or impossibility of a meaningful bonding. Shame can be evoked both by an actual rejection from others and also by inner characterological tendencies to distance oneself from, detach from, overreact to, or destroy relationships. Lansky considered shame the most significant affect in suicidal patient and rated other suicide-related emotional states—such as depression, guilt, psychic pain, and anger—as secondary to the emotional impact of shame. Excessive primitive shame triggered by the experience of incompetence, inadequacy or lack of control can provoke cognitive impairment, autonomic reactions, and self-disintegration. Shame can overwhelm the person with such pain and stress that narcissistic depletion and a state of self-disintegration follow. Narcissistic patients, as shown in the three cases above, can keep separate and unassociated the suicide-related narcissistic or grandiose ideas, on the one hand, and the actual suicidal behavior and its real life-threatening and defeating consequences, on the other. However, once dissociation occurs, the defensive split between grandiose ideas and self-destructive impulses disappears, the self is flooded with primitive shame, and the road is open for life-threatening actions.

Narcissistic rage has usually been associated with grandiosity and increased self-esteem (Kohut, 1977, p. 194), that is, an attempt to protect a narcissistic person's sense of superiority and specialness by depersonalizing or destroying somebody who is experienced as threatening. However, feelings of shame can also motivate anger, rage, or humiliated fury (H. B. Lewis, 1971). The pain of shame and its resulting loss of self-esteem may trigger unfocused anger and hostility (Lindsay-Hartz, 1984; Tangney, Wagner, Fletcher, & Gramzow, 1992; Wicker, Payne, & Morgan, 1983). Such shame-based anger can easily be directed as retaliation toward others, because shame typically involves the imagery of a real or imagined disapproving other. Anger is likely to provide some relief from the global self-condemning and debilitating experience of shame (Tangney et al., 1992). Anger can also be directed toward the self, causing intolerable psychic pain and leading to suicide as a way of escaping such shame-based pain (Baumeister, 1990).

Destructive narcissistic rage or primitive excessive, blind rage reactions have also been associated with functional regression, lack of control, irrationality, and an archaic perception of reality (Kohut, 1972, 1977). Under normal circumstances, shame can have an inhibiting function on aggression and promote a transformation of early rage into mature aggression (Schore 1994). In addition, shame reactions to narcissistic injury, that is, withdrawal, have been seen as opposite to active revengeful narcissistic rage reactions (Kohut, 1972, p. 379). However, the combination of excessive shame and rage can have a mutually magnifying effect leading to explosive, uncontrolled behavior patterns (Schore, 1994). When the grandiose self is threatened, both narcissistic rage and shame erupt. Narcissistic rage, experienced as a loss of control, fuels feelings of shame that further escalates the rage. In the absence of self-protective character structure, the self is then vulnerable to such escalation and to destruction through self-killing.

Assessment and Treatment of Suicidality

Given that suicidal ideations and behavior can occur in patients who are not depressed or whose distress may seem less obvious or even absent to the clinician, the assessment of suicidality should include, in addition to a general exam of mental state, a specific evaluation of suicide risk and of the psychological vulnerability to suicide. Maltsberger (1996) suggested the following risk components to be assessed: (1) past responses to stress, especially losses; (2) vulnerability to three life-threatening affects: aloneness, self-contempt, and murderous rage; (3) the nature and availability of exterior sustaining resources; (4) the emergence and emotional importance of death fantasies; and (5) the patient's capacity for reality testing. For narcissistic patients, it is especially important to pay attention to changes in or losses of resources that are crucial for the patients' self-esteem or sense of specialness, such as work, creativity, special relations, social, financial or professional opportunities or promotions, and so forth. Of special importance is evaluating the patient's ability to identify and tolerate affects and threatening self-experiences, especially a deep sense of worthlessness, inferiority, and shame. As mentioned above, ideas of suicide, and death can harbor narcissistic meanings such as superiority, triumph and revenge or serve to shield against threats. It is also notable that narcissistic patients can be severely suicidal without signs of impaired capacity for reality testing. However, unrealistic grandiose ideas of invulnerability or superiority over life and death, and detachment from one's own body can contribute to psychological disintegration and loss of the capacity to test reality and protect against danger and self-directed rage.

Specific Treatment Considerations

The management and treatment of suicidal narcissistic patients follow the general strategies for treatment of all suicidal patients. A multimodal treatment team approach including both individual and couples or family therapy, psychopharmacological treatment, and hospital or intensive group treatment is usually necessary. Specific suicide consultations and recurrent suicide risk evaluations are recommended as well as the mobilizing of external emotional support systems at work, within the family or close social environment, or through organizations, when appropriate. The immediate goal for the treatment of the acutely suicidal patient is to prevent self-harm or active suicidal behavior. The focus is to help the patient remove him- or herself from or otherwise manage overwhelming intensive experiences and negative feelings. For narcissistic patients who are not overtly depressed, psychopharmacological treatment can be valuable when focusing on acute rage, anxiety, or intolerance of affects. It may at times be difficult to evaluate the urgency and necessity of preventive hospital treatment of the suicidal narcissistic patient because of the patient's tendencies to deny suicide risk, lack overt depressed symptoms, and his or her seemingly high level of reasoning and functioning. A specific consideration is that such patients may react with increased suicidal impulsivity or actual suicidal behavior in response to the suggestion of hospitalization because of experiences of humiliation, loss of control, and social/professional disruption and disgrace triggering feelings of shame and rage. Because suicidality in narcissistic patients often can occur in relation to work- or career-related changes, it may be valuable to include employee assistance program representatives as part of the treatment team. The use of suicide or safety contracts between therapist and patient—that is, an agreement that the patient will not act upon suicidal ideations, and, if not able to follow this agreement, the patient will either page the therapist or go to nearest emergency room—may be useful if a trustful therapeutic alliance is present. However, such contracts may also not be useful as they can create a false idea of a common frame of reference or represent an unrealistic agreement that attempt to shield both the patient's and the treating clinician's reactions (C. M. Miller, Jacobs, & Gutheil, 1998).

Suicidality usually evokes intense feelings in the therapist. Countertransference rage and hatred (Maltsberger & Buie, 1973) can be specifically intense in the treatment of suicidal narcissistic patients. Because such patients tend to provoke hatred by their passive or active attack on the therapist's self-esteem and narcissistic functioning, they easily trigger an urgent sadomasochistic enactment between therapist and patient. In addition, grandiose rescue ambitions can motivate sudden deviations from regular treatment strategies and lead the therapist far away from realistic treatment goals (Gabbard, 2003). The therapist's fear of being abandoned by the patient through suicide is another difficult counter-transference reaction.

There are two types of clinical scenarios with suicidal narcissist patients that are specifically challenging for the therapist. The first relates to situations when acute overt suicidal ideations occur in the context of sudden changes or events in the patient's life that seriously threaten the person's narcissistic balance and grandiose self-image. These include threats to the narcissistic person's view and experience of him- or her-self as capable, competent, and accomplished, such as loss of professional position and capability. They can also involve threats to or loss of a sense of perfectionism, that is, an inability to live up to one's own or others' standards. In fact, several studies support a relationship between perfec-tionism and suicidal ideations in adolescents and college students (Ham-ilton & Schweitzer, 2000; Hewitt, Newton, Flett, & Callander, 1997) and perfectionism and suicidal behavior (successful suicides) in talented and high-achieving people (Apter et al., 1993; Blatt, 1995). Changes or losses of significant, stable sources of narcissistic support or gratification, such as bankruptcies, divorces, lost opportunities for professional promotion/advances, awards, and so forth, are additional such events. These situa-tions can occur gradually or suddenly and be more or less obvious and acutely life-threatening.

Usually, patients in a state of acute suicidal ideation require immedi-ate and multimodal interventions, such as intensive, structured psychiat-ric, psychotherapeutic and psychopharmacological treatment, a mutual agreement between clinician and patient regarding risk evaluation, responsibilities, and communication and an emergency plan. The focus in psychotherapy is, first, to carefully outline and understand the specific narcissistic meaning of the event, that is, the way the event threatened the patient's self-esteem and sense of competence and specialness, and second, to empathically process accompanying feelings of rage, humilia-tion, and shame and possible impulses of revenge or urges for narcissistic control.

It is especially important to explore the occurrence of underlying sadomasochistic impulses in response to such an event. The narcissistic patient tends to capitalize on narcissistic injuries, increase self-loathing, and hold on to the experience of humiliation and feelings of rage. They perpetuate a fantasy of alternating between being a grandiose victim and having superior control and continue to act in a revengeful way through self-defeating or self-destructive suicidal or suicide-related behavior that prevents exploration of new solutions and attitudes that could promote gradual progress. The presence of these dialectical opposites—narcissism and masochism (Cooper, 1989)—sets the stage for escalating suicidal feelings and urges to act self-destructively.

Case vignette

Mr. J had worked for more than 20 years as a vice president together with a female president in a midsize high-tech company. They had over the years managed the company through several crises and changes, with major adjustments to technological advancements and fluctuations in the market economy. Mr. J genuinely and deeply appreciated his boss, and together they had formed a competent and progressive team. After the president's retirement, she was replaced by a shrewd, efficient, and experienced male corporate leader who was specifically chosen to make radical changes to adjust the company to rapidly growing competition from the expanding Asian market. A few months after the shift in executive leadership, Mr. J began feeling depressed. He noted that he was missing his former boss immensely and felt ignored and belittled by his new boss. He found himself sitting and fantasizing at work about various acts of revenge against his new boss. With increased depression, Mr. J believed that he was losing his leadership capacity for the projects he was in charge of. Despite advice from colleagues and family members to look for another job or even to apply to graduate school and get a degree in his special field, Mr. J chose to hold on to his position in the company. However, he felt increasingly humiliated and had recurrent episodes of hostile and revengeful encounters with his new boss. Late one evening, Mr. J made a serious suicide attempt in his office that led to the termination of his position as a vice president for the company. Later, when in psychotherapy, Mr. J admitted that the suicide attempt was intended as revenge toward his new boss and an attempt to interfere with the boss's career. He had also seen it as the only way of removing himself from an utterly humiliating situation. In the continuing psychotherapy, he remembered how he at age 10 when he lost his beloved mother to death from a suddenly developing cancer, he also lost his recently acquired skill to dive. Left with his strict, unemotional, and achievement-focused father, he felt inferior and unable to meet the father's expectations. His previous female boss was like "the good mother who returned" and working under the new boss suddenly brought back images of his strict father.

The second challenging scenario is when the narcissistic persons' suicidal thoughts and ideations remain hidden, even for long periods, or just briefly alluded to without either being acted upon or discussed in depth. This is a scenario that can develop when such ideations are serving to stabilize and/or to increase the patients' self-esteem or protect their sense of self, like a "secret." Suicidal ideations can also be part of a person's affect regulation as a way of processing and mastering unbearable and unavoidable feelings. This adaptive function of suicidality can in fact help to preserve an inner sense of control and coherence, and paradoxically even help the person to stay alive and actively engage in living their lives (Gabbard, 2003).

Case vignette

Mrs. O, a 45-year-old divorced single lawyer, took an overdose of a combination of psychotropic medications and alcohol, with the unwavering determination to kill herself. The action failed but ended in a near-lethal outcome, keeping Mrs. O in a coma for several days. After her divorce 13 years earlier, Mrs. O had devoted 80–90 hours a week to develop a reputable law firm. Her goal was to become no less then the number one lawyer in the region. She wanted to prove to her father that she could succeed in her profession. She also wanted to show that the divorce did not bother her and to prove that her mother was wrong in her negative expectations. Two events drastically interrupted Mrs. O's remarkable career track, first that her firm lost a case that had attracted nationwide attention, and second, that her father unexpectedly died a few weeks after this professional setback. Mrs. O reacted by gradually withdrawing from professional and social life and isolating herself in her home for days, even weeks. At the time of her suicide attempt, Mrs. O was 2 years into psychotherapy, with two sessions each week, but she never revealed to her psychotherapist her initial suicidal ideations or her determined plan to end her life.

Many years later, while in another intensive individual psychotherapy, in which she was more able to speak about the unspeak-
able, Mrs. O revisited the events leading up to her suicide attempt.
She recalled having considered her suicidal plan an entirely private
matter that she was unable to talk about. She did not reveal to the
therapist the part of her life that concerned her feelings about living
and plans to end her life. "It did not even enter my mind," she said,
and she also denied feeling dislike or distrust toward the psychotherapist. Mrs. O recalled that what she had considered a total professional failure combined with the loss of her father, who had been
an exclusive, devoted support for her, made her feel left without
goal or meaning in her life. She felt personally and professionally
crushed and deeply ashamed. She secretly began to fantasize about
a reunion with her father and considered suicide as a way to leave
her overwhelming sense of failure behind and to enter into a better
state together with her deceased father.

This example highlights the complex relationship between affect state
and recalling, and between reactivation and deactivation attachment
modes (Schore, 1994). Studies have shown that retrieval of information
decrease when a person is in a state that differs from the state in which a
particular information or experience was required, and that reactivating
a particular body state is necessary for accessing certain cognitive states
(Bower, 1981; Bower & Gilligan,1979). In other words, the connection
between affect or mood state influences the process of recalling memories and their accompanying psychobiological motivations. With particular relevance for treatment is of course the specific affect or mood the
person is experiencing in the alliance with the therapist/analyst in the
moment that can influence the process of retrieving and recalling. This
is important for understanding and treating people, like Mrs. O, with
chronic and split off suicidal ideations and with serious suicide attempt(s)
in the past, who do not fully engage in the therapeutic alliance. Such
patients may suddenly and surprisingly after years of therapy be able to
recall certain suicidal feelings and cognitive and affect states in the context of a particular transference with the present therapist/analyst. When
treating such patients, the therapist/analyst also have to be aware of and
thoroughly explore the potentially life threatening meaning of certain life
events, such as interrupted careers, that may cause an inner sense of loss

of a control, competence, and capability, which due to intense feelings of shame are withdrawn and kept inaccessible or deactivated in the treatment alliance.

Chronic Suicidality

Chronic suicidal ideations can serve significant narcissistic functions by representing idealized, unrealistic, or omnipotent ideas about ending life and the postdeath states. Suicide can be viewed as something separate and/or different from death and dying, and some people can have the distorted idea that they actually will not die if they kill themselves or that death involve a transformation to a different, better, or higher state (Gerisch, 1998). One woman believed/hoped that she would reunite with her mother. She looked forward to the opportunity to be together with her mother who had died 25 years earlier—not with the deteriorated, ill, and aggressive mother she had known and struggled with, but rather with a healthy, loving mother who had been healed and changed during 25 years in heaven. Another young man (described above) was curious about "life after death" and considered committing suicide to get an opportunity to explore this different state. It added to an image of himself as an unusually innovative and brave scientist and explorer. Some people will talk about committing suicide and dying in very positive idealized terms with positive affects totally unrelated to anguish, despair, and dread. "It will be sssssoooooooo nice, calm, and quiet, I can't wait," said one woman who had made a suicide attempt and remained chronically suicidal for 10 years. It is very easy for the therapist to be seduced into a state of comfort and unrealism with such patients and underestimate both the severity of the suicidality as part of the personality functioning and the risk for acute suicidal behavior. Some people do not want to get rid of their suicidal feelings. "I don't know what I would do if did not feel suicidal," said one patient who had felt chronically suicidal for 25 years.

Self-esteem Regulation in Chronically Suicidal Patients

Suicidal ideations and the awareness of being able to take one's life may be important for a patients self-esteem and his or her sense of dignity and autonomy, even for feeling connected and, in a paradoxical way, providing a sense that it is worth staying alive (Lewin, 1992). The following vignette illustrates such functions.

Case vignette

Mr. S, a divorced man in his mid forties, told his therapist at the first session that he had felt suicidal most of his adult life. He had made three suicide attempts in the past, and nearly succeeded once, but during the past 10 years had not done any harm to himself. Having said that, Mr. S also told the therapist that he presently had suicidal feelings and thoughts several times a week, and he assured the therapist that if things got really bad he would kill himself. This time he said, he would shoot himself with a gun, not try overdosing or any other unreliable procedures.

T: "What makes you feel suicidal?"

Mr. S: "It is this body pain (chronic recurrent pain since a car accident) . . . sometimes it is worse and when the pain gets worse and the painkillers don't help then I begin to feel suicidal, I just want to end it, just end the pain . . ."

T: "So you want to end the pain, but do you actually want to die?"

Mr. S: "Oh . . . no, not really, I just want to get rid of the pain."

T: "And when you think about committing suicide you feel that you can stop the pain?"

Mr. S: "Well . . . If I commit suicide it would be a change . . . I don't really know what would happen to me, but yes . . . I do think that the pain will end . . . And it is always reassuring to know that I can commit suicide if it gets too bad . . ."

T: "It seems to help you to keep yourself in charge of the situation . . ."

Mr. S: "Sort of . . . Yeah . . . I hate when the pain takes over . . . But then . . . I don't want to hurt my wife . . . and I know it would be hard on my kids . . . so that keeps me from doing it . . . But you never know . . . when the pain gets too bad . . . and the painkillers don't work . . . or some other things screw up in my life I might still do it . . ."

T: "Do you think there could be another way than to kill yourself or think about killing yourself?"

Mr. S: "No not as effective . . . I know I can try to distract myself . . . but sometimes I just don't want to . . ."

A few months later Mr. S in session said: "The last few days have been really bad . . . I have felt suicidal every day . . . I was very close this time . . ."

T: "What has happened?"

Mr. S: "Well . . . You see . . . A friend of mine just died."

T: "I am so sorry to hear that."

Mr. S: "Yeah . . . it is weird but I have been thinking that since he died I have to die too, or that I should have died instead of him."

T: "Hmmmmm. Why do you think that?"

Mr. S: "It is a peculiar feeling . . . I don't like that . . . He is gone . . . and I am here . . . I sort of feel guilty . . . or bad . . . I can't stand it . . . Sometimes I think maybe I failed him . . . He got very ill, we all knew it was coming . . . I hated to see him suffer . . . It made me feel horrible . . ."

T: "It can be very painful and overwhelming to lose a close friend."

Mr. S: "I am not good at that . . . The funeral is coming up . . . I hate that too . . . but I suppose I have to go . . . I am supposed to be strong, macho . . . I am a man . . . men don't cry . . . I'd rather just put it aside . . ."

T: "Is that when you feel like killing yourself?"

Mr. S: "Yeah . . . Thinking about suicide is like a relief . . . it makes things feel more bearable . . . I know I can just leave if it becomes too much . . ."

T: "So in other words, feeling suicidal seems to help you replace several other more unbearable feelings, such as feeling like a failure, feeling hatred, feeling dread when having to face something you don't want to face . . ."

Mr. S: "Sort of . . . Yeah . . . As I said . . . it is like a relief . . ."

T : "Is there anything I can do for you?"

Mr. S: "No not really . . . I know you doctors are trying to be helpful, you don't want to see me die . . . but no . . . if it gets too bad I know I should go to the emergency room. Don't get me wrong . . . I do appreciate to talking to you about this . . . But this is between me and myself . . ."

A few sessions later Mr. S said: "I am surprised, but I actually felt better after that time I talked to you about feeling suicidal when my friend had died."

T: "How come, what do you think happened?"

Mr. S: "I am not sure . . . maybe because I can talk to you about suicide without your getting all excited and upset and thinking that I am crazy . . . or thinking you have to hospitalize me . . . I don't belong in the hospital . . . that would make me feel much worse . . . that would really kill me . . ."

T: "I agree with you . . . do you think it was something else that made you feel better . . ."

Mr. S: "Not really . . . [Silence] Well I am not really used to talking about my real feelings . . . It feels kind of embarrassing . . . Maybe . . . I don't know . . . that could have made a difference . . ."

Comment

Suicidal ideations helped Mr. S to feel control over his uncontrollable physical pain. Suicidal ideations were also the preferred method of control for Mr. S because he was not really interested in practicing other methods of controlling or distracting himself from his pain. In other words, Mr. S regulated his pain by thinking about suicide. In addition, Mr. S regulated both self-esteem and his affects with a suicidal preoccupation that replaced stressful overwhelming and/or intolerable but normal feelings. His preoccupation with suicide was specifically related to feelings of rage/hatred, inferiority, and shame. He hated himself when he could not master and control physical and emotional pain. He also hated himself when he felt inferior, like a failure, or controlled by others or outside circumstances. In addition, he felt ashamed of his real feelings, but surprisingly not of feeling suicidal. In terms of the intersubjective dynamics in relationship to the therapist, Mr. S had expected to evoke strong feelings and responses from the therapist that could serve to deflect attention from his own inner feelings by being labeled as "crazy." By focusing on exploring Mr. S's suicidal ideations in depth and outlining their occurrence and functioning, the therapist encouraged Mr. S active participation and capacity for self-reflection.

Several features in Mr. S's personality and functioning contributed to his ability to commit himself to treatment and to be able to explore and gradually detach himself from his suicidal ideations. First of all, Mr. S wanted to take responsibility for his suicidality, and he presented the emergency plan if feeling acutely at risk for suicidal behavior. In addition, he was attached and committed to his family and did not want to cause suffering. Nevertheless, Mr. S did not want to involve the therapist; he wanted to keep her informed but at arm's length, and he needed to remain in control on his own terms. The therapist understood that Mr. S did not aim at manipulating her and sensed that maintaining the therapeutic alliance and discussing the context and purpose of Mr. S's suicidal feelings was of highest priority. The aim was to help Mr. S to translate and transform suicidal ideations and impulses into interpersonal and affective experiences, especially as they related to distrust, hatred, revenge, and inferiority. As Mr. S was gradually more able to tolerate and discuss his feelings, his preoccupation with suicide came to an end. In other words, Mr. S no longer needed suicidality as a self-regulator.

Conclusions

Suicidal behavior in narcissistic patients can be understood as an effort to avoid facing a major shameful defeat, loss, or narcissistic injury. Many narcissistic patients do not think of killing themselves. The denial and rationalization of the suicide-related or suicidal behavior seem to represent a narcissistic defense against the acknowledgment of such conditions. Often there is a fantasy system connected to the grandiose self-experience, usually infiltrated with aggressive impulses and controlling or revengeful strivings. These narcissistic fantasies not only help detach the suicidal act from its true meaning (death) but also add narcissistic meanings (as mentioned above) to the suicidal behavior or the state of being dead. These considerations make evaluations of suicidal states in narcissistic patients especially challenging.

8

Correction or Corrosion?

Changes in Pathological Narcissism

This chapter explores the nature of changes in pathological narcissism, focusing specifically on changes instigated not through therapeutic interventions but through life events that the individual has experienced as either corrective or corrosive. Such experiences can contribute to a modification or transformation of narcissism, with specific character traits and interpersonal and behavioral patterns ceasing to have pathological narcissistic functions (Ronningstam, Gundersen, & Lyons, 1995). However, life events can also contribute to an increase in pathological narcissism and the development of trauma-associated narcissistic symptoms (Simon, 2000), severe NPD, or even a psychotic disorder with delusional grandiosity. The relationship between such external events and the work that takes place within the therapeutic alliance between patient and therapist or analyst may be complex and less obvious. The question is whether corrective life experiences that promote structural change and improved interpersonal relations actually may lessen the motivation for pursuing treatment. Such experiences can in themselves support a progressive and more satisfying involvement in life in ways that are experienced as less threatening to the self-esteem than involvement in intensive psychotherapy. On the other hand, an acute or gradual increase in pathological narcissism following a corrosive life event may actually motivate a person to seek treatment and work toward personal change.

Changeability in Pathological Narcissism

People with narcissistic personalities have long been considered resistant to change. Absence of overt symptoms, denial of problems and limitations, and perpetuating self-enhancing behavior decrease their motivation for change. Because the etiology of pathological narcissism stems from interactional patterns and self-regulatory failures during early childhood (P. Kernberg, 1989, 1998; Schore, 1994), it is considered to be an ego-syntonic and stable disorder with deeply ingrained personality patterns. In addition, a recent twin study (Torgersen et al., 2000) reported a strong genetic influence for NPD (79%), suggesting that heritability plays a major role in the development of NPD. Moreover, psychological studies of self-esteem regulation have confirmed that people with a high degree of narcissism have high but unstable self-esteem. They have a pronounced sensitivity to critical evaluations and intense anger and hostility in reaction to perceived threats to more favorable self-images (Rhodewalt & Morf, 1998). Continuous search for affirmation of the grandiose but vulnerable self and interpersonal self-regulatory strategies that actually tend to undermine the self and prevent integration of positive feedback (Morf & Rhodewalt, 2001) are both features of the narcissistic personality that hinder change and personal growth.

Another obstacle stems from narcissistic individuals' specific resistance to seeking treatment. They usually do not identify or experience their character traits as problematic. Circumstances and relationships that support or enhance grandiosity or seal specific narcissistic vulnerabilities may further convince them that they function well. The treatment process in itself requires capacities that may be impaired or absent in the narcissistic person, that is, capacity for symbolization and tolerance of mutual interpersonal relationships. Once in treatment, narcissistic patients may experience the setting and interaction as provocative, humiliating, or meaningless. The narcissistic need for excessive admiration was associated with discontinuing of psychotherapy (Hilsenroth, Castlebury, & Blais 1998), indicating another explanation for the reluctance to and disinterest in treatment. In addition, the relationship with the therapist activates intolerable feelings such as generalized psychic pain (O. Kernberg, 1993a), rage, inferiority, shame, and envy. The narcissistic patient's capacity to commit to and benefit from a long-term therapeutic alliance may be limited due to low affect tolerance and an urge to destroy what the other person has and what may be possible to receive.

Clinical accounts report on narcissistic patients' tendencies to maintain their distance by secretly compartmentalizing and "dosageing" information on their own terms, by holding on to their own hidden agendas vis-à-vis the therapist, by rejecting interpretations, and by refusing to discuss issues relevant to their problems and treatment progress. They describe experiencing contact with a psychotherapist as intrusive or demeaning, as evidence of their own imperfection or failure, or even as threatening, and they use strategies to protect self-esteem and avoid intolerable affects such as pain, rage, shame and envy, or inferiority and helplessness.

Changes Within Treatment

Freud's suggestion that people with narcissistic neuroses were not candidates for psychoanalysis because they could not develop transference remained unchallenged for several decades. However, modern object relational, self-psychological, and interpersonal approaches to pathological narcissism have spurred increasing optimism regarding the treatability and prognosis of people with narcissistic disorders. Two psychoanalytic strategies have proved effective: One, suggested by O. Kernberg (1975, 1984), relies heavily on reality testing and confrontation and interpretation of the pathological grandiose self and the negative transference. The other approach, developed by Kohut (1966, 1971, 1977), focuses on empathic observations and the development and working through of three types of transference—mirroring, idealizing, and twinship or alter ego transference (Ornstein, 1998)—as a way of correcting the structural deficits that characterize narcissistic disorders. A third, less well-known strategy (Fiscalini, 1993; Fiscalini & Grey, 1994) uses a method of active interpersonal coparticipant psychoanalytic inquiry, which alternates between confrontational and empathic exploration of the narcissistic transference–countertransference matrix. This strategy focuses on the patient's difficulties in tolerating challenges to subjective perspectives and self-esteem, while actively engaging the patient in an exploration of interpersonal interactions.

Explorations and a new understanding of psychic change (Horowitz, Kernberg, & Weinshel, 1993) have had specific relevance for the treatment of narcissistic disorders. Applicable to NPD is new understanding of transference and countertransference development and of projective identification and enactment (Renik, 1993, 1998), combined with a broadened scope of therapeutic interventions (Stewart, 1990). Several recent clinical reports have documented advances in the treatment of narcissistic disorders as the therapist/analyst acknowledged enactment and countertransference (Bateman, 1998; Glasser, 1992; Ivey, 1999; Jørstad, 2001; O. Kernberg, 1999). In addition, treatment modalities other than psychoanalysis and psychoanalytic psychotherapy may also be efficient in modifying maladaptive features of NPD. The most promising is the schema-focused therapy (Young, 1998), which combines cognitive, behavioral, experiential, and transference-based techniques to change schema modes.

Changes Outside Treatment

In addition to these observations of change within the therapeutic setting, changes in narcissistic people have been noted outside treatment, in the context of personal development and life events. O. Kernberg (1980) pointed to the narcissistic patient's capacity to learn from experiences and to develop more self-awareness over time. He noted that the potential for change might increase in middle age as people face their limitations as well as more severe or long-term consequences of their narcissistic personality and lifestyle. A capacity to mourn and to tolerate the experience of depression, including guilt and regret, indicate a better prognosis. Kohut (1968) noted that changes take place in the narcissistic personality throughout the life cycle via compensation for narcissistic vulnerability and deficiencies and via transformations of narcissistic strivings such as grandiosity and exhibitionism.

In a follow-up study of patients diagnosed with NPD (Ronningstam & Gunderson, 1996; Ronningstam, Gunderson, & Lyons, 1995), we found a significant decrease in the level of pathological narcissism over a 3-year period. The characteristics of the treatment (i.e., length, type and intensity) were relatively equally distributed among those who improved and those who did not. Surprisingly, in the follow-up interview the patients who had improved considered their changes primarily the result of life events and not of treatment. An analysis of patients' accounts of life events suggested that a decrease in pathological narcissism was related to three kinds of corrective life experiences: achievements, new durable relationships, and disappointments or disillusionments. In other words, our study suggests that factors and circumstances outside treatment—actual life events and the patient's specific experience of such events—contribute to change in people with NPD.

Corrective Life Events

The idea that experiences in themselves can be corrective was first proposed by Alexander (Alexander & French, 1946), who applied the term "corrective emotional experience" to experiences within psychotherapy. While studies of the impact of life events (G. W. Brown & Harris, 1989) usually have focused on the corrosive effect of stressful experiences, no previous studies have explored the idea that life events may have a corrective impact. The three corrective experiences we identified in the follow-up interviews were (1) corrective achievements, (2) corrective interpersonal relationships, and (3) corrective disillusionment.

Achievements, such as graduations or receipt of an award or acceptance in a sought-for position, school, or program, were the most common corrective life events in our study. They contributed to a better balance among ambitions, ideals, and fantasies and inner goals, leading to a more accepted, realistic sense of self, with less defensive grandiosity and narcissistic reactions. Indeed, achievements could promote a noticeable transformation, as the experience of attaining goals and successfully managing responsibilities and collaborations replaced feelings of being underestimated and misunderstood, as well as arrogance and feelings of contempt and envy.

Interpersonal relationships—those that involved a commitment to a long-term, intimate connection with another person—also reduced pathological narcissism. Within the context of such a relationship, the narcissistic sense of specialness and superior isolation was replaced by the experience of mutual specialness and engagement, with diminished feelings of contempt and devaluation and less entitled and exploitative behavior. The capacity to maintain a close, mutual relationship turned out to be crucial for sustained change. It involved a test of the person's tolerance of affects, and closeness may activate unbearable feelings such as pain, rage, resentment, envy, and/or shame, which can make continuing commitment impossible.

Corrective disillusionment involved experiences that challenged the person's previous sense of grandiosity but led to an adjustment of the self-concept that was more in accord with the person's actual capabilities. Such adjustments involved recognizing of personal, intellectual, and/or vocational limitations and of unrealistic expectations or lost opportunities (Ronningstam & Gunderson, 1996). Corrective disillusionment can develop from the experience of major losses or restrictions in life such as career interruptions (see below) or from corrosive life events that disrupt or severely challenge customary ways of regulating affects and self-esteem. Paradoxically, such disillusionment can also develop in the context of advancements and new personal and professional responsibilities. However, if such experiences are too severe, traumatic, or disruptive, or if they occur in the absence of support, they may lead to chronic grandiose disillusionment and a worsening of pathological narcissism.

Interpersonal Relativeness—The Avenue to Change

Further analysis of our results showed that what might appear to be enduring pathological narcissism can actually include both a changeable context-dependent type of pathological narcissism and a stable NPD. A higher level of pathological narcissism in the area of interpersonal relations, especially an inability to be involved in committed long-term relationships and intense reactiveness to criticism and defeats, indicated a more severe and enduring form of NPD. We also found that narcissistic pathology in the area of self-esteem regulation (i.e., grandiosity and a sense of superiority) changed considerably over a 3-year period, suggesting that this aspect of pathological narcissism may be more context dependent and susceptible to change. The most important changes were in the realm of interpersonal relations. Patients were in general less contemptuous, devaluating, entitled, and exploitative than they had been 3 years earlier. Surprisingly, however, there was no difference in treatment experiences between patients with an enduring long-term NPD and those whose narcissistic pathology diminished.

Our results suggest that those who have a more severely impaired capacity for interpersonal relationships, including difficulties in making long-term commitments and intense reactions to defeat and criticism from others, are less capable of changing and improving over time. In other words, the presence of these narcissistic problems is significantly associated with poor prognoses and absence of change, and hence indicates more enduring forms of NPD (Ronningstam, Gunderson, & Lyons, 1995). In contrast, those whose narcissistic pathology is primarily related to self-esteem regulation or affect regulation, with less severe impairment in the capacity to form and maintain intimate relationships, have better prognosis, and are more able to change.

Corrosive Life Events

In our study of group treatment for people whose careers had been interrupted by the onset of a major mental illness, that is, depressive disorder, bipolar disorder, posttraumatic stress disorder, or an escalating personality disorder (Ronningstam & Anick, 2001), we found that the experience of narcissistic humiliation was central for people whose lives and self-esteem had been focused on professional activities (see also chapter 6 this volume). Strong reactions—especially shame and rage—to the career interruption were notable in most of the participants. Retrospectively, for several of the group members their symptoms may be diagnosed as trauma-associated narcissistic symptoms (Simon, 2001), which occur as a traumatic stressor overwhelms the self and trigger symptoms such as shame, humiliation and rage. The nature of this type of trauma was usually more interactional and experienced as a personal attack or insult compared to traumas leading to posttraumatic stress disorder.

However, events that would be considered potentially corrective of narcissistic pathology may also in certain cases lead to increased pathological narcissism. For some people with more severe pathological narcissism or NPD, evidence of their actual achievements may challenge specific aspects of narcissism related to exhibitionism, shame, guilt, and entitlement. For example, one woman was a financial planner whose 15-year career had involved several successful accomplishments and rewards, as well as several unsuccessful attempts to advance toward top executive positions with increased responsibilities, influence, and salary. After having been bypassed in an important promotion, her career was interrupted by a severe depression and a serious suicide attempt. She revealed that with each actual success and promotion, she used to have an immediate reaction of entitlement, aggressively demanding higher positions and rewards, with strong feelings of emptiness and boredom, loss of interest in the work itself and in the company, and an unrealistically evaluation of her contribution and experience. Her supervisors pointed out that although she was capable of extremely good work with projects and customers, she tended to perform inconsistently, misjudged situations, became agitated, and lacked leadership skills and a full understanding of the company's mission. For this woman, actual achievements, recognitions, and rewards were paradoxically experienced as humiliating reminders and evidence of her limitations, not of her capability. Self-critical comparisons of herself with colleagues resulted in anger, resentment, envy, and self-pity that precluded opportunities for professional growth and feelings of pride.

Case Vignettes

The following case vignettes illustrate how life events may contribute to changes in pathological narcissism. The first two of these patients were seen in once- or twice-weekly long-term individual psychotherapy when the corrective life events occurred. Although both psychotherapies were focused toward change, primarily by addressing losses and regulation of rage and impulsivity, it is the author's belief that the noticeable accompanying changes the patients presented were highly influenced by the occurrence of each specific event. The patients' own conceptualizations and interpretations of the events seemed to represent active independent efforts toward self-regulation and self-control that constructively influenced their motivation toward progressive changes in behavior and life functioning. These efforts also seemed to represent changes in the patients' interactive balance between pathological and healthier narcissistic functioning.

The first case vignette illustrates how gradual change in life context combined with a specific life event suddenly led to major improvement in the patient's narcissistic disorder. The second case describes on how a patient's interpretation of a specific sudden life event contributed to a rapid major change in his severe narcissistic disorder. The third case discusses a major increase in pathological narcissism with development of severe trauma-associated narcissistic symptoms after an extremely corrosive life event.

"My horrible neighbors cured my revengefulness"

Mr. H, a man in his late thirties, sought psychotherapy after having been fired from his job as an insurance sales representative. Despite being a capable and intelligent man who had had periods of successful and appreciated professional contributions, this was one of numerous jobs he had lost or left in a state of rage and frustration in the past 15 years. The reasons for the job losses had been Mr. H's tendencies to get into verbal fights with peers, colleagues, and supervisors. In addition, he had for many years had serious arguments with his neighbors, whom he described as provocative and uneducated. He felt superior as he mobilized his talents in verbal argumentation, and he felt entitled to get back at people because of what he experienced as their impoliteness, stupidity, sarcasm, non-cooperativeness, or opposition of him. He described feeling a certain thrilling excitement as the arguments and animosity escalated, and he could exercise his power and expose his superior talents in what he considered "verbal assassination." The arguments also provided Mr. H with an opportunity for self-righteous complaints about their never-ending efforts to terrorize him and make his life miserable.

The difficult experiences in the context of the latest job loss convinced Mr. H that he needed to seek help. Despite the therapist's persistent attempts to explore, clarify, and interpret Mr. H's motives for engaging in these interactions, as well as the disadvantages and risks involved, Mr. H did not want to give them up. Neither did the therapist's attempts to explore the specific narcissistic feelings and behavior involved, such as superiority, hostility, revengeful-ness, entitlement, risk-taking, and a sadomasochistic oscillation between victimization and persecution, help to change Mr. H's behavior. Instead, Mr. H took pride in the belief that he could actu-ally end these continuing conflicts with his neighbors on his own terms whenever he wanted, just by ignoring or being polite to his neighbors, but he considered it his choice when that would hap-pen. Puzzled and frustrated by Mr. H's steadfast attachment to this pattern, the therapist felt as if she was being kept at arm's length from Mr. H's actual life experiences, since he came to the sessions providing only small doses of information about his whereabouts, and often overwhelmed the therapist with complaints and detailed, agitated descriptions of past and present hostile interactions.

However, over a period of 6 years of treatment in psychotherapy that involved exploration of many hostile and threatening experi-ences during Mr. H's first 12 years of life, a number of important changes took place. Mr. H became engaged to a woman whose commitment and loyalty exceeded his recurrent attempts to esca-late conflicts and end relationships; he became a father, and he was accepted to a prestigious business school. One day he showed up in his therapist's office and said with a big smile, "My horrible neigh-bors cured my revengefulness." After a specifically nasty and threat-ening encounter with the neighbors, Mr. H had, to his own surprise, begun to feel more burdened, uncomfortable, and threatened by his neighbors and less compelled to participate in verbal fights. He actually found his behavior deviant, especially in the context of his new educational pursuits. He noticed that the excitement he had previously experienced when arguing with his neighbors was fading, and he realized that these encounters could potentially be harmful to his daughter and detrimental to his future career in business. However, as he found that he was less able than he thought to control the course of the interactions by acting reasonable and polite toward his neighbors or by ignoring provocative comments, he and his family decided to move to a friendlier neighborhood.

Obviously Mr. H's hostile, superior and revengeful behavior in his relationships with neighbors and colleagues ceased to serve a narcissistic function. Instead, Mr. H's energy and ambitions were gradually redirected toward more adapted and mature goals that better served adjusted narcissistic functions of self-regard, parental responsibility, and progress toward career goals. The question remains, however, what actually contributed to the change in Mr. H's attitudes and behavior? Mr. H's capacity to engage in long-term relationships with the therapist, with his fiancée and mother of his daughter, and with his daughter clearly helped form the foundation and motivation for change in his pathological narcissistic patterns. Being accepted to and pursuing an educational program that would lead to a professional career modified Mr. H's narcissistic pursuits as well as his self-esteem and affect regulation. Aggressive, revengeful exhibitionism was replaced by professional ambitions and achievements. It may be that Mr. H had to develop more adjusted ego goals and aspirations before he could alter his pathological narcissistic patterns. Mr. H believed that the actual realizations and experiences that brought about an identifiable change in his narcissistic behavior occurred outside the psychotherapy. The question is whether the motivational and emotional processes involved in experiencing a life event and coming to a realization through such an event were necessary conditions for creating noticeable structural changes in Mr. H. The question is also in what way the psychotherapy by focusing on more distant but also more original experiences addressed important aspects of self-esteem and interpersonal competence that paved the way for changes in Mr. H's personal life. Or could it be that fully acknowledging the interaction with the psychotherapist and the specific transference vis-à-vis her would have triggered intolerable feelings of dependency, fear of rejection, rage, and envy?

"It was a gift from God . . ."

Mr. J was in his mid forties, married with four children, and an owner of a successful industrial development company. He was a shrewd, arrogant, independent man. Although he usually felt proud and capable, he had also throughout his adult life struggled with an unspecific sense of inferiority because he was short and had false teeth. He had chosen to marry a woman from a third-world country because he considered himself dependable and believed he would be able to provide well for her.

After nearly 20 years of married life, Mr. J became suspicious that his wife was having an affair. Finding evidence, Mr. J experienced a peculiar combination of shock, severe humiliation, and sexual excitement. After a few months he decided to take action. In a state of impaired judgment, partial denial of the reality and consequences of the events happening to him, and feelings of humiliation, entitlement, and self-righteousness, Mr. J began making a series of devastating decisions. First, he decided to talk to his wife's family, hoping to get their support. Instead, they believed that Mr. J had violated his wife's integrity and rejected his appeal. After a few sessions of couple therapy, his wife requested a divorce. Because Mr. J believed he was not at fault, he failed to plan carefully for his own legal representation in the divorce while his wife found representation by a very skilled divorce attorney. After a year, Mr. J had to sign a divorce agreement in which he lost most of his assets and had to assume substantial financial responsibility for his children and ex-wife. In addition, believing that "nothing bad can happen to me after all this," Mr. J made a series of miscalculations and risky maneuvers in his business and soon had to file for bankruptcy. He made numerous unsuccessful attempts to get back into work after he closed his business. Although professionally competent with several promising opportunities for advanced positions or start-ups of new business, Mr. J was for a long time either too depressed or apathetic to work or too critical, scornful, and prone to attacks of rage and conflicts with bosses and colleagues. He had great difficulty tolerating peers and subordinating himself to others. Mr. J began to envy and despise people who worked successfully, and former business partners and colleagues gradually began to avoid him.

At this point, Mr. J was advised by a relative to seek psychiatric help, since he suffered from insomnia and felt confused, desperate, depressed, suicidal, and apathetic and struggled with severe rage. Mr. J, who despised subordination and helplessness and had always taken pride in being "sane" and self-sufficient, considered psychiatric treatment extremely humiliating and the ultimate evidence of his own failure and incompetence. The first clinician he consulted refused to continue treatment after a few weeks, finding Mr. J too arrogant, noncompliant, and derogative of his profession and competence. The second clinician, after a few months of treatment, became concerned about Mr. J's murderous rage and decided to report his concerns, resulting in him being fired by Mr. J. The third clinician found Mr. J to be a desperate, severely humiliated man who had murderous, revengeful narcissistic rage toward his former wife. The divorce and events leading up to it had apparently escalated a pre-existing narcissistic condition of entitlement and masochism, as well as an extreme vulnerability in self-esteem and proneness to intense reactivity, including rage and vengefulness. Mr. J also suffered from partially impaired reality testing and severe impairments both in self-regard and in the capacity to protect and defend himself. He was also oblivious to the consequences of his own feelings and actions and how he himself contributed to worsening his situation. He felt that he had been caught by an evil destiny and that whatever he did, his situation worsened. Although Mr. J did not believe in treatment, he nevertheless felt compelled to pursue psychotherapy and he faithfully attended the sessions. He saw the psychotherapist at worst as an unpredictable enemy, and at best as a helpless and incompetent creature at the bottom of the societal totem pole. As such, however, Mr. J did obviously not consider the therapist as threatening. On the contrary, Mr. J conveyed a paradoxical sympathy for the therapist who had to attend to his miseries. The psychotherapy, which lasted for one and a half years, was complicated by the fact that Mr. J was not a man of insight or self-reflection. He was concrete and action oriented, and for a long time he resented and resisted most treatment interventions. However, he had no history of criminal or dangerous behavior, and he did indeed adhere to the therapist's request to get a lawyer to help him with his legal matters.

During the first phase of the treatment, Mr. J was mainly preoccupied with discussing his rage toward his ex-wife and his murderous, revengeful, homicidal wishes toward her. The therapist oscillated between feeling forced into either a position as an ally in a murder conspiracy or a position of a magic guardian protecting Mr. J from his own rage. Gradually, Mr. J's reality anchoring improved as he began to realize that he was not capable of killing his ex-wife (i.e., that he had murderous rage but was not a murderer). Although Mr. J had never been an actively religious person, he reached out for a higher power and began to pray to God, asking that God take his former wife's life through an accident or illness. As his appeals remained unfulfilled Mr. J felt paralyzed, became severely depressed and increasingly suicidal, and was at that point in such serious financial difficulty that he was at risk of becoming homeless. He refused psychopharmacological treatment with an antidepressant, and after a consultation, the therapist suggested electroconvulsive therapy. Mr. J promised to consider this over the weekend.

During that weekend, a friend of Mr. J invited him to a type of evangelic meeting, during which he entered a state of ecstasy and fainted. Shortly after this event, Mr. J got a job selling home appliances in a small but progressive company. Despite denying his spirituality or religiousness, he was convinced that this job was a special gift from God. Mr. J found his new work appealing and worthwhile. He got along well with his supervisors and colleagues; he put in long hours and began to get commissions. His life turned around and he gained self-esteem, began feeling valued and competent, reported feeling cautiously hopeful, and developed new interests and friendships. His depression lifted and his feelings toward his former wife changed from murderous rage to quietly controlled resentment and hatred. His capacity to assume his role and responsibilities as a father improved. His scornful aggressiveness toward other people diminished, and he felt increasingly capable of pursuing and fulfilling professional and personal goals. Because of his work schedule, he attended psychotherapy sessions less frequently and finally stopped treatment without any formal termination.

A series of severely corrosive and traumatic events activated a murder-ous narcissistic rage in Mr. J. In the psychotherapy, this rage was gradually internalized and transformed into depression and directed toward himself in intense suicidal ideations. The corrective life event—a new job that allowed him to regain his capacity to work and earn money—occurred in the context of a serious financial and self-destructive threat to his life. It also occurred in response to a narcissistic interpretation of this event. To perceive a job opportunity as "a gift from God" was apparently a way that Mr. J could tolerate dependency, accept help and still feel special, and be able to give up the old narcissistic pattern of aggressive, superior independence. The question remains how Mr. J's experience of ecstasy in the context of the therapist's recommendation of electroconvulsive therapy contributed to the transformation of his pathological narcissism into healthier interpersonal relationships and interactions and vocational pursuits.

"I was facing something that was stronger than me . . . "

Mr. C, a married man in his late forties, was the chief supervisor of an airport traffic control tower at an air base in a foreign coun-try. He had many years of experiences and was considered skilled and reliable. As a young man he had joined the air force intending to become a pilot, but because of a physical limitation had been unable to pursue that career track and had chosen to become a traf-fic controller instead. He reported feeling great enthusiasm about his work. He specifically took pride in having landed thousands of airplanes, including jumbo jets and huge cargo planes, without accidents or other complications. In addition, he openly described himself as the person who independently and single-handedly brought down the airplanes, as if the pilots were not involved in the landing operation. One day, the weather conditions were unpredict-able, and during a landing procedure that Mr. C was supervising, the aircraft suddenly lost direction and crashed, and 25 people lost their lives. In the extensive and detailed investigation that fol-lowed, Mr. C's professional judgment, conduct, and management of the events prior to and during the accident were found to have met professional standards, and he was not held responsible for the accident. However, during the investigation Mr. C developed a sustained fantasy (Zelin et al., 1983) that he could have prevented the accident by using an alternative strategy for landing the plane. He was convinced that because he was found not responsible for the accident, he was the only one who knew about this alternative strategy and that he alone could have decided to use it but had chosen not to do so. Although Mr. C received substantial professional support and returned to work soon after the initial investigation was completed, he experienced increasing difficulty in concentrating and performing his professional tasks.

Exploration during a brief psychotherapy consultation a couple of years after the accident revealed that Mr. C continued to be preoccupied with the fantasy of preventing the plane crash. He spent several hours a day reviewing, second by second, the events and decisions leading up to the accident, and in his fantasy he used the secret and imaginative alternative landing strategy, which he believed could have prevented the accident. In his inner world, he felt in control and as strong and capable as he had felt during his entire professional life. Externally, he was struggling with overwhelming feelings of inferiority and failure. He repeatedly stated, "I was facing something that was stronger than me—Nature! That has never happened to me before." He denied feeling guilty or believing that he had caused the accident. Neither was he able to show concerns about the 25 people who died and their families. However, he began suffering from depressed mood with severe impulsive outbursts of rage, irritability, chronic suicidality, and homicidal ideations. Neuropsychological testing indicated a long-term limitation in the capacity for abstract thinking and for understanding abstract contexts and relations. Despite intensive treatment, Mr. C did not improve, mainly because he encapsulated himself in an effort to prove his own competence. He felt totally alone and out of reach of all other human beings. What kept him alive seemed to be his own internal self-appraisal.

This is an example of an extreme worsening of pathological narcissism in the context of a seriously traumatic and corrosive life event that severely challenged the patient's experience of himself as capable, worthy, and superior. The experience led to a dramatic increase in symptoms of pathological narcissism, especially delusional grandiosity and self-persecutory attacks, accompanied by severe symptoms of posttraumatic stress disorder. It also exacerbated a pre-existing narcissistic condition and triggered trauma-associated narcissistic symptoms. Mr. C had compensated for his interrupted plans to become a pilot by believing that he indeed *was* the pilot and the only one in charge during the landing procedure, a fantasy that apparently had supported his professional self-esteem and sense of capability for a long time without interfering with his capacity to perform his professional duties. However, after the accident, it seems that this compensatory pathological narcissistic constellation prevented full reality testing and engagement in a therapeutic alliance.

Conclusions

Pathological narcissism is not a static, fixed state of psychopathology. On the contrary, the interchange between stability and changeability and the oscillation and interaction between healthy and pathological narcissism constitute an active ongoing process both within each person and in his or her relationships and life context. A planned or unexpected life event and its specific narcissistic meaning can either augment self-esteem and promote personal growth or lead to an increased sense of inferiority, with accompanying defensive grandiosity, interpersonal aggressiveness, and detachment. Our research has shown that pathological narcissism can decrease over time through corrective life events, even independently of treatment. Our studies have also shown that pathological narcissism can increase as a reaction to corrosive experiences that threaten or disrupt the individual's self-experience and normal self-regulation. In some cases when the corrosive event is experienced as traumatic and specifically threatening to underlying narcissistic vulnerability, the increase in pathological narcissism can represent trauma-associated narcissistic symptoms. Further clinical and empirical studies of the complexity of narcissism are called for, specifically studies focusing on factors influencing motivation for change and patterns of interactions that promote change in psychotherapy with the narcissistic patient.

Epilogue

People with narcissistic disorders have long been considered difficult to understand and treat. As they usually are provocative, demanding, controlling and entitled they evoke negative feelings and challenging countertransference reactions in those who treat them (Malin, 1990). On the other hand, they can also be seemingly engaged and compliant in long-term treatment without noticeable changes occurring. Clinicians are usually puzzled by and generally reluctant to take on narcissistic people as interpersonal conflicts and treatment failures are more common than not. The long history of the diagnosis of narcissistic personality disorder (NPD) within psychoanalysis and psychodynamic psychology and psychiatry has accumulated valuable clinical observations and encouraging treatment efforts. Nevertheless, the absence of a comprehensive empirical database, that can guide our understanding of these patients, is still a significant obstacle for developing a clinically useful model and realistic treatment guidelines for narcissistic personality functioning.

This volume has described evidence supporting the core features of pathological narcissism and narcissistic disorder, such as grandiosity and self-esteem fluctuations, shame, intense reactivity to criticism, and expressions of aggression ranging from arrogant, haughty behavior and interpersonal control and hostility to overt rage and violent reactions. Fewer observations and evidence are available to clarify the nature of impaired empathic capacity, inability to form long-term interpersonal commitments, envy, and entitlement. The regulatory model for narcissism, as suggested in chapter 4, aims to organize and integrate narcissistic functioning in a dimensional perspective. The vicissitudes between

normal and pathological narcissism, high and low self-esteem, affect dysregulation with predominance of aggression versus shame, high and low
moral functioning, overt reactive and/or covert inhibited interpersonal
patterns are accounted for, as are the three types of prototypic personality disorders: the shy, arrogant and psychopathic.

The question remains whether NPD primarily is a self-esteem disorder, an affect regulation disorder, a mood or temperament disorder, a
cognitive disorder, and/or a combination of some or all of the above. The
answer to this question bears significant treatment implications. Future
explorations of the core and nature of narcissistic functioning may indicate the advantage of a multimodal approach to understanding and cure
that takes into consideration the nature of narcissism as well as the specific obstacles and difficulties that the narcissistic individual encounters
when seeking treatment and attempting to change. Narcissism certainly
invites continuing integrative efforts of inquiry and change from psychoanalytic, developmental psychological, psychopharmacological, dynamic
psychiatric, cognitive, and psychosocial learning perspectives.

Advances in neuroscience have opened new perspectives on the interaction between genes and environment in personality development and
on the influence of neurological correlates on emotional and interpersonal
regulation. This is of specific importance for understanding narcissistic
functioning (Kaplan Solms, Solms, 2000) especially such central features
as impaired empathic functioning (Eslinger, 1998; Preston de Waal, 2002),
proneness to and intolerance of shame (Schore, 1998), hypersensitivity
and reactivity, interpersonal hostility, and fluctuations in self-esteem. The
suggestion that effective psychotherapy leading to long-term personality changes also influences brain functioning and causes changes in gene
expression and anatomical pattern in the brain (Kandel, 1998) can be
highly relevant. Is it possible that narcissistic patients' treatment resistance and the seemingly ego-syntonic nature of narcissistic functioning
may be further understood in the context of specific neurobiological and
neuropsychological patterns?

New advances in psychoanalytic treatment have focused on the challenges involved in treating severely disturbed people with chronic anger,
envy, resentment, and tendencies to reject and destroy relationships to
others—including those trying to help them (Bateman, 1998; Cohen
2003; Ivey 1999; Jørstad, 2001). The discussions among traditional and
relational psychoanalysts have specifically focused on the value of the
therapist's/analyst's acknowledgment, understanding, and tolerance of

their own strong negative affects vis-à-vis such patients (Cohen, 2002). Efforts have focused on maintaining the therapeutic alliance through such affect storms and discussing the affects in depth with the patients. Efforts have also focused on persistently and non-judgmentally helping patients to understand the origins and function of their affects in the enactment in the therapeutic alliance. This is of significant relevance as it can help those treating narcissistic patients to avoid their own detachment from or moral judgment of the patient, or their affect attacks and criticism, and/or the premature termination of treatment due to their anger and disappointment in the patient's low ability to relate and progress. It may be possible that further studies of the mutually participating interaction between therapist/analyst and the narcissistic patient, combined with appreciation of the narcissistic patients' real and actual capability to understand, interact and change, can raise new hopes both for people with narcissistic disorders and those who treat them.

Few disorders are the target of such negative criticism, blame, hostility, and misunderstanding as NPD. It is my hope that a deeper and more thorough understanding of the complexity of narcissism and narcissistic functioning can help to promote the development of flexible and integrated treatment strategies in the future. More knowledge and awareness among those living or working with, and those treating narcissistic individuals can raise motivation for their challenging efforts to change. It is my foremost hope that narcissistic people themselves, who struggle with concealed inner suffering, devastating interpersonal conflicts and isolation, can gain the courage and willingness to seek treatment and work toward optimal changes.

Appendix

A.1. Diagnostic criteria for 301.81: narcissistic personality disorder from *DSM-IV* and *DSM-IV-TR*

A pervasive pattern of grandiosity (in fantasy or behavior), need for admiration, and lack of empathy, beginning in early adulthood and present in a variety of contexts, as indicated by five (or more) of the following:

1. Has grandiose sense of self-importance (e.g., exaggerates achievement and talents, expects to be recognized as superior without commensurate achievements)
2. Is preoccupied with fantasies of unlimited success, power, brilliance, beauty, or ideal love
3. Believes that he or she is "special" and unique and can only be understood by, or should be associated with, other special or high-status people (or institutions)
4. Requires excessive admiration
5. Has a sense of entitlement, i.e., unreasonable expectations of especially favorable treatment or automatic compliance with his or her expectations
6. Is interpersonally exploitive, i.e., takes advantage of others to achieve his or her own ends
7. Lacks empathy; is unwilling to recognize or identify with the feelings and needs of others
8. Is often envious of others or believes that others are envious of him or her
9. Shows arrogant, haughty behaviors or attitudes

A.2. Diagnostic Interview for Narcissism (DIN), Second Edition.

Grandiosity (3-year framework)

1. The person exaggerates talents, capacity and achievements in an unrealistic way.* ‡ †
2. The person believes in his/her invulnerability or does not recognize his/her limitations.
3. The person has grandiose fantasies.* ‡ †
4. The person believes that he/she does not need other people.
5. The person regards himself as unique or special compared with other people.* ‡ †
6. The person regards himself/herself as generally superior to other people. †
7. The person behaves self-centeredly and/or self-referentially. †
8. The person appears or behaves in a boastful or pretentious way. †

Interpersonal Relations (3-year framework)

9. The person has a strong need for admiring attention. * ‡ †
10. The person unrealistically idealized other people.
11. The person devalues other people including feelings of contempt.
12. The person has recurrent and/or deep feelings of envy toward other people.* ‡
13. The person reports or behaves entitled, i.e., has unreasonable expectations of favors or other special treatment.* ‡ †
14. The person appears or behaves in condescending, arrogant, or haughty ways. ‡ †
15. The person is exploitative, i.e., takes advantage of or uses other people. * ‡
16. The person lacks empathy (is unable both to understand and to feel for other people's experiences).* ‡
17. The person has been unable to make close, lasting emotional commitments to others.

Reactiveness (3-year framework)

18. The person is hypersensitive.

19. The person has had unusually intense feelings in response to criticism or defeat.*
20. The person has behaved or felt suicidal or self-destructive in response to criticisms or defeat.
21. The person has reacted with inappropriate anger in response to criticism or defeat.
22. The person has hostile, suspicious reactions in response to the perception of others' envy. †

Affects and mood states (1-year framework)
23. The person has deep, sustained feelings of hollowness.
24. The person has deep, sustained feelings of boredom.
25. The person has deep, sustained feelings of meaninglessness.
26. The person has deep, sustained feelings of futility.
27. The person has deep, sustained feelings of badness.

Social and Moral adaptation (5-years framework)
28. The person has been capable of high school/work achievement (academic, employment, creative) †
29. The person has superficial and changing values and interests.
30. The person shows a disregard for usual/conventional values or rules of society.
31. The person has broken laws one or a few times under circumstances of being enraged or as a means to avoid defeat.
32. The person has recurrent antisocial behavior.
33. The person's sexual behavior includes perversions, promiscuity, and/or a lack of inhibitions.

---

* DSM-III-R criteria for narcissistic personality disorder.
‡ DSM-IV criteria for narcissistic personality disorder.
† Discriminating features for NPD (Ronningstam & Gunderson, 1991)
Source: Gunderson J. & Ronningstam E. McLean Hospital, Belmont, MA, 1990.

References

Abrams, D. M. (1993). Pathological narcissism in an eight-year-old boy: An example of Bellak's T.A.T. and C.A.T. diagnostic system. *Psychological Psychology, 10*(4), 473–591.

Adler, G. (1981). The borderline-narcissistic personality disorder continuum. *American Journal of Psychiatry, 138*(1), 46–50.

Akhtar, S. (1988). Hypomanic personality disorder. *Integrative Psychiatry, 6*, 37–52.

Akhtar, S. (1989). Narcissistic personality disorder: Descriptive features and differential diagnosis. *Psychiatric Clinics of North America,12*(3), 505–530.

Akhtar, S. (1992). Broken structures: Severe personality disorders and their treatment. Northvale, NJ: Jason Aronson.

Akhtar, S. (1997, May). *The shy narcissist.* Paper presented at the 150th American Psychiatric Association annual meeting, San Diego, CA.

Akhtar, S. (2003). *New clinical realms. Pushing the envelope of theory and technique.* Northvale, NJ: Jason Aronson.

Akiskal, H. S. (1992). Delineating irritable and hyperthymic variants of the cyclothymic temperament. *Journal of Personality Disorders, 6*(4), 326–342.

Akiskal, H. S., & G. Mallya. (1987). Criteria for the "soft" bipolar spectrum: Treatment implications. *Psychopharmacology Bulletin, 23*, 68–73.

Aleksandrowicz, D. R. (1980). Psychoanalytic studies of mania. In R. Belmaker & H. M. Van Praag (Eds.), *Mania—an evolving concept* (pp. 309–322). Utrecht: MTP.

Alexander, F., & French, T. M. (1946). *Psychoanalytic therapy: principles and applications.* Oxford, England: Ronald Press.

Alonso, A., & S. Rutan. (1988). The treatment of shame and the restoration of self-respect in groups. *International Journal of Group Psychotherapy, 38*(1), 3–14.

Alonso, A., & S. Rutan. (1993). Character change in group therapy. *International Journal of Group Psychotherapy, 43*(4), 439–51.

American Psychiatric Association. (1994). *Diagnostic and statistical manual of mental disorders* (4th ed.). Washington, DC: Author.

American Psychiatric Association. (2000). *Diagnostic and statistical manual of mental disorders* (4th ed., text revision). Washington, DC: Author.

Apter, A., A. Bleich, R. King, S. Kron, A. Fluch, M. Kotler, & Cohen, D. J. (1993). Death without warning? A clinical postmortem study of suicide in, 43 Israeli adolescent males. *Archives of General Psychiatry, 50,* 138–142.

Arns, P., & J. Linney. (1993). Work, self and life satisfaction for persons with severe and persistent mental disorders. *Psychosocial Rehabilitation Journal, 17*(20), 63–79.

Attwood, T. (1998). *Asperger's syndrome. A guide for parents and professionals.* London: Jessica Kingsley Publishers.

Axelrod, S. (1999). *Work and the evolving self. Theoretical and clinical considerations.* Hillsdale, NJ: Analytic Press.

Bach, S. (1975). Narcissism, continuity and the uncanny. *International Journal of Psychoanalysis, 56,* 77–86.

Bach, S. (1977a). On narcissistic fantasies. *International Review of Psychoanalysis, 4,* 281–293.

Bach, S. (1977b). On the narcissistic state of consciousness. *International Journal of Psychoanalysis, 58,* 209–233.

Bach, S. (1985). *Narcissistic states and the therapeutic process.* New York: Jason Aronson.

Balint, M. (1959). Distance in space and time. In *Thrills and regression.* New York: International Universities Press.

Barth, F. D. (1988). The role of self-esteem in the experience of envy. *American Journal of Psychoanalysis, 48*(3), 198–210.

Basch, M. F. (1983). Empathic understanding: A review of the concept and some theoretical considerations. *Journal of the American Psychoanalytic Association, 31*(1), 101–126.

Bateman, A. (1998). Thick- and thin-skinned organizations and enactment in borderline and narcissistic disorders. *International Journal of Psychoanalysis, 79,* 13–25.

Baumeister, R. F. (1990). Suicide as escape from self. *Psychological Review, 97*(1), 90–113.

Baumeister, R. F., T. F. Heatheron, & D. M. Tice. (1993). When ego threats lead to self-regulation failure: Negative consequences of high self-esteem. *Journal of Personality and Social Psychology, 64*(1), 141–156.

Baumeister, R. F., L. Smart, & J. M. Boden. (1996). Relation of threatened ego-tism to violence and aggression: The dark side of high self-esteem. *Psychological Review, 103*, 5–33.

Beck, A. T., A. Freeman, & Associates (1990). *Cognitive therapy of personality disorders.* New York: Guilford Press.

Berezin, M. A. (1977). Normal psychology of the aging process, revisited—II. The fate of narcissism in old age, clinical case reports. *Geriatric Psychiatry, 10*, 9–26.

Berglas, S. (1986). *The success syndrome: Hitting the bottom when you reach the top.* New York: Plenum Press.

Berglas, S. (2002). The very real dangers of executive coaching. *Harvard Business Review, 80*(6), 86–92.

Bergman, I. (1987). *Laterna magica.* Stockholm: Norstedts.

Berkowitz, D. A., R. L. Shapiro, J. Zinner, & E. R. Shapiro. (1974a). Concurrent family treatment of narcissistic disorders in adolescence. *International Journal of Psychoanalytic Psychotherapy, 3*(4), 379–396.

Berkowitz, D. A., R. L. Shapiro, J. Zinner, & E. R. Shapiro. (1974b). Family con-tributions to narcissistic disturbances in adolescents. *International Review of Psychoanalysis, 1*, 353–362.

Black, D. W., G. Warrack, & G. Winkur. (1985). The Iowa record linkage study. Suicides and accidental deaths among psychiatric patients. *Archives of General Psychiatry, 42*, 71–74.

Blais, M. A., M. J. Hilsenroth, & F. D. Castlebury. (1997). Content validity of the *DSM-IV* borderline and narcissistic personality disorder criteria sets. *Comprehensive Psychiatry, 38*(1), 31–37.

Blatt, S. J. (1995). The destructiveness of perfectionism. *American Psychologist, 50*(12), 1003–1020.

Bleiberg E. (1994). Normal and pathological narcissism in adolescence. *American Journal of Psychotherapy, 48*(1), 30–51.

Bodlund, O., L. Ekselius, & E. Lindström. (1993). Personality traits and disor-ders among psychiatric outpatients and normal subjects on the basis of the SCID screen questionnaire. *Nordisk Psychiatrisk Tidskrift, 47*, 425–433.

Book, H. E. (2002). How leadership and organizational structure can create a winning corporate culture. In J. P. Kahn & A. M. Langlieb (Eds.), *Mental health and productivity in the workplace: A handbook for organizations and clinicians* (pp. 205–232). New York: Jossey-Bass.

Bourgeois, J. A., R. M. Crosby, M. J. Hall, & K. G. Drexler. (1993). An examina-tion of narcissistic personality traits as seen in a military population. *Military Medicine, 158*(3), 170–174.

Bower, G. H. (1981). Mood and memory. *American Psychologist, 36*, 129–148.

Bower, G. H., & S. G. Gilligan. (1979). Remembering information related to one self. *Journal of Research in Personality, 13*, 420–432.

Brieger, P., U. Ehrt, & A. Marneros. (2003). Frequency of comorbid personality disorders in bipolar and unipolar affective disorders. *Comprehensive Psychiatry, 44*(1), 28–34.

Bronish, T. (1996). The relationship between suicidality and depression. *Archives of Suicide Research, 2*, 235–254.

Broucek, F. J. (1982). Shame and its relationship to early narcissistic developments. *International Journal of Psychoanalysis, 63*, 369–378.

Brown, G. W., & T. O. Harris (Eds.). (1989). *Life events and illness.* New York: Guilford Press.

Brown, N. W. (2001). *Children of the self-absorbed.* Oakland, CA: New Harbinger Publications.

Brown, N. W. (2002). *Working with the self-absorbed.* Oakland, CA: New Harbinger Publications.

Burney, J., & H. J. Irwin. (2000). Shame and guilt in women with eating disorder symptomatology. *Journal of Clinical Psychology, 56*, 51–61.

Bursten, B. (1973). Some narcissistic personality types. *International Journal of Psychoanalysis, 54*, 287–300.

Bushman, B. J., & R. F. Baumeister. (1998). Threatened egotism, narcissism, self-esteem, and direct and displaced aggression: Do self-love or self-hate lead to violence? *Journal of Personality and Social Psychology, 75*(1), 219–229.

Campbell, W. K., G. D. Reeder, C. Sedikides, & A. J. Elliot. (2000). Narcissism and comparative self-enhancement strategies. *Journal of Research in Personality, 34*, 329–347.

Charles, M. (2001). Stealing beauty: An exploration of maternal narcissism. *Psychoanalytic Review, 88*(4), 549–570.

Chasseguet-Smirgel, J. (1985). *Creativity and perversions.* New York: Norton.

Clark, L. P. (1926). The phantasy method of analyzing narcissistic neurosis. *Psychoanalytic Review, 13*, 225–232.

Cohen, S. (1988). Super-ego aspects of entitlement (in rigid characters). *Journal of American Psychoanalytic Association, 38*, 409–427.

Cohen, S. (2002). *Affect intolerance in patient and analyst.* Northvale, NJ: Jason Aronson.

Cohen, S. (2003). The thrall of the negative and how to analyze it. *Journal of the American Psychoanalytic Association, 51* (2): 465–489.

Cooper, A. M. (1981). Narcissism. In S. Areti, H. Keith, & H. Brodie (Eds.), *American handbook of psychiatry* (Vol. 4, pp. 297–316). New York: Basic Books.

Cooper, A. M. (1988). The narcissistic-masochistic character. In R. A. Glick & I. D. Meyers (Eds.), *Masochism. Current psychoanalytic perspectives* (pp. 117–138). Hillsdale, NJ: American Psychoanalytic Press.

Cooper, A. M. (1989). Narcissism and masochism. *Psychiatric Clinics of North America, 12*(3), 541–552.

Cooper, A. M. (1998). Further developments of the diagnosis of narcissistic personality disorder. In E. Ronningstam (Ed.), *Disorders of narcissism: Diagnostic, clinical, and empirical implications* (pp. 53–74). Washington, DC: American Psychiatric Press.

Cooper, A. M., & E. Ronningstam. (1992). Narcissistic personality disorder. In A. Tasman & M. Riba (Eds.), *American Psychiatric Press review of psychiatry* (Vol. 11, pp. 80–97). Washington, DC: American Psychiatric Press.

Cording, C., & B. Huebner Liebermann. (2000). Chronishe Suizidalität im Spiegel der psychiatrischen Basisdokumentation. *Krankenhausepsychiatrie, 11*, 582–585.

Crosby, R. M., & M. J. Hall. (1992). Psychiatric evaluation of self-referred and non-self-referred active duty military members. *Military Medicine, 157*, 224–229.

Dahl, A. (1998). Psychopathy and psychiatric comorbidity. In T. Millon, E. Simonsen, M. Birket-Smith, & R. Davis (Eds.), *Psychopathy: Antisocial, criminal and violent behavior* (pp. 291–303). New York: Guilford Press.

Dali, S. (1937). *Metamorphose de narcisse*. Paris: Editions Surrealistes. (rept. and trans. as *Metamorphosis of Narcissus*. New York: Julien Levy)

de la Barca, P. C. (1976). Eko och Narcissus [Eco y Narciso; trans. (from Spanish) R. Hallqvist]. Uddevalla, Sweden: Bokförlaget Trevi (Original work published 1661)

Dodes, L. M. (1990). Addiction, helplessness and narcissistic rage. *Psychoanalytic Quarterly, 59*, 398–419.

Dolan-Sewell, R. T., R. F. Krueger, & M. T. Shea. (2001). Co-occurrence with syndrome disorders. In W. L. Livesley (Ed.), *Handbook of personality disorders. Theory, research and treatment* (pp. 84–104). New York: Guilford Press.

Donaldson-Pressman, S., & R. M. Pressman. (1994). *The narcissistic family— diagnosis and treatment*. San Francisco: Jossey-Bass.

Dowson, J. H. (1992). *DSM-III-R* narcissistic personality disorder evaluated by patients' and informants' self-report questionnaires: Relationship with other personality disorders and a sense of entitlement as an indicator of narcissism. *Comprehensive Psychiatry, 33*(6), 397–406.

Elkind, D. (1991). Instrumental narcissism in parents. *Bulletin of Menninger Clinic, 55*, 299–307.

Ellis, H. (1898). Auto-erotism: A psychological study. *Alienist and Neurologist, 19*, 260–299.

Ellis, H. (1928). The conception of narcissism. In H. Ellis, *Studies in the psychology of sex: Vol. 7. Eonism and other supplementary studies* (pp. 347–375). Philadelphia: F. A. Davis Company.

Emmons, R. A. (1981). Relationship between narcissism and sensation seeking. *Psychological Report, 48,* 247–250.

Emmons, R. A. (1984). Factor analysis and construct validation of the narcissistic personality inventory. *Journal of Personality Assessment, 48,* 291–300.

Emmons, R. A. (1987). Narcissism: Theory and measurement. *Journal of Personality and Social Psychology, 52*(1), 11–17.

Eslinger, P. J. (1998). Neurological and neuropsychological bases of empathy. *European Neurology, 39,* 193–199.

Etchegoyen, H. R., M. L. Benito, & M. Rabih. (1987). On envy and how to interpret it. *International Journal of Psychoanalysis, 68,* 49–61.

Etzersdorfer, E. (2001, August). *The psychoanalytical positions on suicidality in german speaking regions.* Paper presented at the International Congress on Suicidality and Psychoanalysis, Hamburg, Germany.

Fairbairn, W. R. D. (1952). *An objects relation theory of the personality.* New York: Basic Books.

Fava, M., J. E. Alpert, J. S. Borus, A. A. Nierenberg, J. A. Pava, & J. F. Rosenbaum. (1996). Patterns of personality disorder comorbidity in early-onset versus late-onset major depression. *American Journal of Psychiatry, 153*(10), 1308–1312.

Fava, M., A. H. Farabaugh, A. H. Sickinger, E. Wright, J. E. Alpert, S. Sonawalla, A. A. Nierenberg, & T. T. Worthington. (2002). Personality disorders and depression. *Psychological Medicine, 32*(6), 1049–1057.

Fava, M., & J. F. Rosenbaum. (1998). Anger attacks in depression. *Depression and Anxiety, 8*(Suppl. 1), 59–63.

Fee, R. L., & J. P. Tangny. (2000). Procastination: A means of avoiding shame or guilt? *Journal of Social Behavior and Personality, 15*(5), 167–184.

Fenichel, O. (1945). *The psychoanalytic theory of neurosis.* New York: Norton.

Ferenczi, S. (1980). *First contribution to psychoanalysis.* New York: Brunner/Mazel. (Original work published 1913)

Fernando, J. (1998). The etiology of narcissistic personality disorder. *The Psychoanalytic Study of the Child, 53,* 141–158.

Feshbach, N. D. (1975). *Empathy in children,* Some theoretical and empirical considerations. *Counseling Psychologist, 5,* 25–30.

Fiscalini, J. (1994). Narcissism and coparticipant inquiry—explorations in contemporary interpersonal psychoanalysis. *Contemporary Psychoanalysis, 30*(4), 747–776.

Fiscalini, J., & A. Grey. (1993). *Narcissism and the interpersonal self.* New York: Columbia University Press.

Fonagy, P. (1993). Aggression and the psychological self. *International Journal of Psychoanalysis, 74,* 471–485.

Fonagy, P. (1999). Attachment, the development of the self and its pathology in personality disorders. In J. Derksen, C. Maffei, & H. Groen (Eds.), *Treatment of personality disorders* (pp. 53–68). New York: Kluwer Academic/Plenum.

Fonagy, P. (2001). *Attachment theory and psychoanalysis.* New York: Other Press.

Fonagy, P., G. Gergely, E. L. Jurist, & M. Target. (2002). *Affect regulation, mentalization, and the development of the self.* New York: Other Press.

Freud, S. (1957). Three essays on the theory of sexuality. In J. Strachey (Ed. & Trans.), *The standard edition of the complete psychological works of Sigmund Freud* (Vol. 7, pp. 125–243). London: Hogarth Press. (Original work published 1905)

Freud, S. (1957). Psychoanalytic notes on an autobiographical account of a case of paranoia. In J. Strachey (Ed. & Trans.), *The standard edition of the complete psychological works of Sigmund Freud* (Vol. 12, pp. 9–82). London: Hogarth Press. (Original work published 1911)

Freud, S. (1957). On narcissism. In J. Strachey (Ed. & Trans.), *The standard edition of the complete psychological works of Sigmund Freud* (Vol. 14, pp. 66–102). London: Hogarth Press. (Original work published 1914)

Freud, S. (1957). Instincts and their vicissitudes. In J. Strachey (Ed. & Trans.), *The standard edition of the complete psychological works of Sigmund Freud* (Vol. 14, pp. 109–140). London: Hogarth Press. (Original work published 1915)

Freud, S. (1957). Metapsychological supplement to the theory of dreams. In J. Strachey (Ed. & Trans.), *The standard edition of the complete psychological works of Sigmund Freud* (Vol. 14, pp. 217–235). London: Hogarth Press. (Original work published 1917)

Freud, S. (1957). Libidinal types. In J. Strachey (Ed. & Trans.), *The standard edition of the complete psychological works of Sigmund Freud* (Vol. 21, pp. 217–220). London: Hogarth Press (Original work published 1931)

Gabbard, G. (1979). Stage fright. *International Journal of Psychoanalysis, 60,* 383–392.

Gabbard, G. (1983). Further contributions to the understanding of stage fright: Narcissistic issues. *Journal of the American Psychoanalytic Association, 31,* 423–441.

Gabbard, G. O. (1989). Two subtypes of narcissistic personality disorder. *Bulletin of the Menninger Clinic, 53,* 527–532.

Gabbard, G. (1997). The vicissitudes of shame in stage fright. In C. W. Socarides & S. Kramer (Eds.), *Work and its inhibitions: Psychoanalytic essays* (pp. 209–220). Madison, CT: International Universities Press.

Gabbard, G. O. (2003). Miscarriages of psychoanalytic treatment with suicidal patients. *International Journal of Psychoanalysis, 84,* 249–261.

212   References

Gabbard, G. O., & S. W. Twemlow. (1994). The role of mother-son incest in the pathogenesis of narcissistic personality disorder. *Journal of the American Psychoanalytic Association, 42*(1), 171–189.

Gacono, C. B., J. R. Meloy, & J. L. Berg. (1992). Object relations, defensive operations, and affective states in narcissistic, borderline and antisocial personality disorders. *Journal of Personality Assessment, 59*(1), 32–49.

Gacono, C. B., J. R. Meloy, & T. R. Heaven. (1990). A Rorschach investigation of narcissism and hysteria in antisocial personality. *Journal of Personality Assessment, 55*(1/2), 270–279.

Garber, B. (1989). Deficits in empathy in the learning disabled child. In K. Filed, B. Cohler, & G. Wool (Eds.), *Learning and education: Psychoanalytic perspectives* (pp. 617–635). Madison, CT: International Universities Press.

Garber, B. (1991). Analysis of a learning disabled child. In *The annual of psychoanalysis (A publication of the Institute of Psychoanalysis).* (Vol. 19, pp. 127–150). Hillsdale, NJ: Analytic Press.

Gerisch, B. (1998). "This is not death, it is something safer": A psychodynamic approach to Sylvia Plath. *Death Studies, 22,* 735–761.

Gibson, I. (1997). *The shameful life of Salvador Dali.* New York: Norton.

Giovaccini, P. (2000). *Impact of narcissism.* Northvale, NJ: Jason Aronson.

Glad, B. (2002). Why tyrants go too far: Malignant narcissism and absolute power. *Political Psychology, 23*(1), 1–37.

Glasser, M. (1992). Problems in the psychoanalysis of certain narcissistic disorders. *International Journal of Psychoanalysis, 73,* 493–503.

Glickauf-Hughes, C., & M. Wells. (1995). Narcissistic characters with obsessive features: Diagnostic and treatment considerations. *The American Journal of Psychoanalysis, 55*(2), 129–143.

Goldberg, A. (1973). Psychotherapy of narcissistic injuries. *Archive of General Psychiatry, 28,* 722–726.

Golomb, M., M. Fava, M. Abraham, & J. F. Rosenbaum. (1995). Gender differences in personality disorders. *American Journal of Psychiatry, 154*(4), 579–582.

Goodsitt, A. (1985). Self psychology and the treatment of anorexia nervosa. In D. M. Garner & P. E. Garfinkel (Eds.), *Handbook of psychotherapy for anorexia nervosa and bulimia* (pp. 55–87). New York: Guilford Press.

Gramzow, R., & J. P. Tangney. (1992). Proneness to shame and the narcissistic personality. *Personality & Social Psychology Bulletin, 18*(3), 369–376.

Gran, U. (1976). Förord [Foreword]. In Calderon de la Barca, *Eko och Narcissus* [in Swedish; trans. (from Spanish) Eco y Narciso] (pp. 5–10). Uddevalla, Sweden: Bokförlaget Trevi.

Greenwald, D. F., & D. W. Harder. (1998). Domains of shame. Evolutionary, cultural, and psychotherpeutic aspects. In P. Gilbert & B. Andrews (Eds.),

Shame: Interpersonal behavior, psychopathology and culture (pp. 225–245). New York: Oxford University Press.

Groopman, L. C., & A. M. Cooper. (1995). Narcissistic personality disorder. In G. O. Gabbard (Ed.), *Treatments of psychiatric disorders* (2nd ed., pp. 2327–2343). Washington, DC: American Psychiatric Press.

Grothstein, J. S. (1984a). A proposed revision of the psychoanalytic concept of primitive mental states: Part II. The borderline syndrome—section 2. The phenomenology of the borderline syndrome. *Contemporary Psychoanalysis, 20*, 77–119.

Grothstein, J. S. (1984b). A proposed revision of the psychoanalytic concept of primitive mental states: Part II. The borderline syndrome—section 3. Disorders of autistic safety and symbiotic relatedness. *Contemporary Psychoanalysis, 20*, 266–343.

Grundberger, B. (1971). *Narcissism: Psychoanalytic essays*. New York: International Universities Press.

Guile, J. M., L. Sayegh, L. Bergeron, H. Fortier, D. Golberg, & J. Gunderson. (2004). Initial reliability of the diagnostic interview for narcissism adapted for preadolescents: Parent version (P-DIN). *Journal of Canadian Child and Adolescent Psychiatry Review, 13*(3), 73–79.

Gunderson, J. (1984). *Borderline personality disorder*. Washington, DC: American Psychiatric Press.

Gunderson, J. (2001). *Borderline personality disorder. A clinical guide*. Washington, DC: American Psychiatric Publishing.

Gunderson, J.G., L.C. Morey, R.L. Stout, A.E. Skodol, M.T. Shea, T.H. McGlashan, M.C. Zanarini, C.M. Grilo, C.A. Sanislow, S. Yen, M.T. Daversa, & D.S. Bender. (2004). Major depressive disorder and borderline personality disorderd revisited: Longitudinal interactions. *Journal of Clinical Psychiatry, 65*(8), 1049–1056.

Gunderson, J., & M. E. Ridolfi. (2001). Borderline personality disorder. Suicidality and self-mutilation. In H. Hendin & T. Mann (Eds.), *Annals of New York Academy of Sciences*, Vol. 932, pp. 61–77.

Gunderson, J., & E. Ronningstam. (2001). Differentiating antisocial and narcissistic personality disorder. *Journal of Personality Disorders, 15*(2), 103–109.

Gunderson, J., E. Ronningstam, & A. Bodkin. (1990). The diagnostic interview for narcissistic patients. *Archives of General Psychiatry, 47*, 676–680.

Gunderson, J., E. Ronningstam, & L. Smith. (1991). Narcissistic personality disorder: A review of data on *DSM-III-R* descriptions. *Journal of Personality Disorder, 5*, 167–177.

Gunderson, J., E. Ronningstam, & L. Smith. (1996). Narcissistic personality disorder. In T. Widiger, A. Frances, H. A. Pincus, R. Ross, M. First, & W. Wake-field-Davis (Eds.), *DSM-IV sourcebook* (Vol. 2, pp. 745–756). Washington, DC: American Psychiatric Association.

Guntrip, H. (1969). *Schizoid phenomena, object relations and self.* New York: International Universities Press.

Habimana, E., & L. Masse. (2000). Envy manifestations and personality disorders. *European Psychiatry, 15*(Suppl. 1), 15–21.

Hamilton, T. K., & R. D. Schweitzer. (2000). The cost of being perfect: Perfectionism and suicide ideations in university students. *Australian & New Zealand Journal of Psychiatry, 34*(5), 829–835.

Hansen, P. W., A. G. Wang, K. B. Stage, & P. Kragh-Sorensen. (2003). Comorbid personality disorder predicts suicide after major depression: A 10-year follow-up. *Acta Psychiatrica Scandinavica, 107*(6), 436–40.

Harpur, T.J., A. R. Hakstian, & R.D. Hare. (1988). Factor structure of the psychopathy checklist. *Journal of Consulting and Clinical Psychology, 56,* 741–747.

Harpur, T. J., R. D. Hare, & A. R. Hakstian. (1989). A two-factor conceptualization of psychopathy: Construct validity and implications for assessment. *Psychological Assessment: A Journal of Consulting and Clinical Psychology, 1,* 6–17.

Hart, S. D., & R. D. Hare. (1998). The association between psychopathy and narcissism—theoretical views and empirical evidence. In E. Ronningstam (Ed.), *Disorders of narcissism: Diagnostic, clinical and empirical implications* (pp. 415–436). Washington, DC: American Psychiatric Press.

Hartman, H. (1964). *Essays on ego psychology.* New York: International Universities Press.

Hartocollis, P. (1980). Affective disturbances in borderline and narcissistic patients. *Bulletin of the Menninger Clinic, 44,* 135–146.

Hassan, R. (1995). *Suicide explained.* Victoria: Melbourne University Press.

Hastings, M. E., L. Northman, & J. P. Tangney. (2000). Shame, guilt and suicide. In T. Joiner & D. Rudd (Eds.), *Suicide science—expanding the boundaries* (pp. 67–79). Boston: Kluwer Academic Publishers.

Havens, L. (1993). The concept of narcissistic interactions. In J. Fiscalini & A. Grey (Eds.), *Narcissism and the interpersonal self* (pp. 189–199). New York: Columbia University Press.

Henseler, H. (1974). *Narzisstische Krisen. Zur Psychodynamik des Selbstmordes.* Opladen, Germany: Westdeutcher Verlag.

Henseler, H. (1981). Psychoanalytische Theorien zur Suizidalitaet. In H. Henseler & C. Reimer (Eds.), *Selbstmordgefardung. Zur Psychodynamik und Psychotherapie* (pp. 113–135). Stuttgart: Frommann-Holzboog.

Henseler, H. (1991). Narcissism as a form of relationship. In J. Sandler, E. S. Person, & P. Fonagy (Eds.), *Freud's "On Narcissism: An Introduction"* (pp. 195–215). New Haven, CT: Yale University Press.

Hewitt, P. L., & G. L. Flett. (1991). Perfectionism in the self and social contexts: Conceptualization, assessment, and association with psychopathology. *Journal of Personality and Social Psychology, 60*(3), 456–470.

Hewitt, P. L., J. Newton, G. L. Flett, & L. Callander. (1997). Perfectionism and suicide ideations in adolescent psychiatric patients. *Journal of Abnormal Child Psychology, 25*(2), 95–101.

Hibbard, S. (1992). Narcissism, shame, masochism, and object relations: An exploratory correlational study. *Psychoanalytic Psychology, 9*, 489–508.

Hilsenroth, M. J., F. D. Castlebury, & M. A. Blais. (1998). The effects of *DSM-IV* cluster B personality disorder symptoms on the termination and continuation of psychotherapy. *Psychotherapy, 35*(2), 163–176.

Hilsenroth, M. J., J. C. Fowler, J. R. Padawer, & L. Handler. (1997). Narcissism in the Rorschach revisited: Some reflections on empirical data. *Psychological Assessment, 9*(2), 113–121.

Hilsenroth, M. J., L. Handler, & M. A. Blais. (1996). Assessment of narcissistic personality disorder: A multi-method review. *Clinical Psychology Review, 16*(7), 655–693.

Hilsenroth, M. J., S. R. Hibbard, M. R. Nash, & L. Handler. (1993). A Rorschach study of narcissism, defense, and aggression in borderline, narcissistic and cluster C personality disorders. *Journal of Personality Assessment, 60*, 346–361.

Hogan, C. (1983a). Psychodynamics. In P. Wilson (Ed.), *Fear of being fat* (pp. 115–128). New York: Jason Aronson.

Hogan, C. (1983b). Object relations. In P. Wilson (Ed.), *Fear of being fat* (pp. 129–149). New York: Jason Aronson.

Hogan, C. (1983c). Transference. In P. Wilson (Ed.), *Fear of being fat* (pp. 153–168). New York: Jason Aronson.

Holdwick, D. J., M. J. Hilsenroth, F. D. Castlebury, & M. A. Blais. (1998). Identifying the unique and common characteristics among the *DSM-IV* antisocial, borderline and narcissistic personality disorder. *Comprehensive Psychiatry, 39*(5), 277–286.

Hollender, M. H. (1965). Perfectionism. *Comprehensive Psychiatry, 6*, 94–103.

Horney, K. (1939). *New ways in psychoanalysis.* New York: Norton.

Horowitz, M. J. (1975). Sliding meanings: A defense against threat in narcissistic personalities. *International Journal of Psychoanalytic Psychotherapy, 4*, 167–180.

Horowitz, M. J., O. Kernberg, & E. M. Weinshel (Eds.). (1993). *Psychic structure and psychic change. Essays in honor of Robert S. Wallerstein.* Madison, CT: International Universities Press.

Houston, K., K. Hawton, & R. Shepperd. (2001). Suicide in young people aged 15–24: A psychological autopsy study. *Journal of Affective Disorders, 63* (1–3), 159–170.

Hunt, W. (1995). The diffident narcissist: A character-type illustrated in *The Beast in the Jungle* by Henry James. *International Journal of Psychoanalysis, 76*, 1257–1267.

Imbesi, L. (2000). On the etiology of narcissistic personality disorder. *Issues in Psychoanalytic Psychology, 22*(2), 43– 58.

Ivey, G. (1999). Transference-countertransference constellations and enactments in the psychotherapy of destructive narcissism. *British Journal of Medical Psychology, 72*, 63–74.

Jacobson, E. (1964). *The self and the object world.* New York: International Universities Press.

Jang, K. L., W. J. Livesley, P. A. Vernon, & D. N. Jackson. (1996). Heritability of personality disorder traits: A twin study. *Acta Psychiatrica Scandinavica, 94*, 438–444.

Joffe, R., & J. Regan. (1988). Personality and depression. *Journal of Psychiatric Research, 22*, 279–286.

Johnson, J. G., P. Cohen, E. Smailes, S. Kasen, J. M. Oldham, A. E. Skodol, et al. (2000). Adolescent personality disorders associated with violence and criminal behavior during adolescence and early adulthood. *American Journal of Psychiatry, 157*, 1406–1412.

John, O. P., & R. W. Robins. (1994). Accuracy and bias in self-perception: Individual differences in self-enhancement and the role of narcissism. *Journal of Personality and Social Psychology, 66*(1), 206–219.

Johnson, C., & M. E. Connors. (1987). *The etiology and treatment of bulimia nervosa.* New York: Basic Books.

Johnson, W. (1995). Narcissistic personality as a mediating variable in manifestations of post-traumatic stress disorder. *Military Medicine, 160*(1), 40–41.

Johnsson-Fridell, E., A. Öjehagen, & L. Träskman-Bendz. (1996). A 5-year follow-up study of suicide attempts. *Acta Psychiatrica Scandinavica, 93*, 151–157.

Jones, E. (1913). The god complex. In E. Jones (Ed.), *Essays in applied psychoanalysis* (Vol. 2, pp. 244–265). London: Hogarth Press.

Jørstad, J. (2001). Avoiding unbearable pain. Resistance and defense in the psychoanalysis of a man with a narcissistic personality disorder. *Scandinavian Psychoanalytic Review, 24*, 34–45.

Kandel, E. (1998). A new intellectual framework for psychiatry. *American Journal of Psychiatry, 155*(4), 457–469.

Kaplan Solms, K., & M. Solms. (2000). *Clinical studies in neuro-psychoanalysis.* London: Karnac Books.

Karlsson, E. (1977). *Barn och Sorg. En studie kring sorgearbete under barndomen* [Children and mourning. A study of bereavement in childhood]. Stockholm: Natur och Kultur.

Kates, N., B. Greiff, & D. Hagen. (1990). *The psychosocial impact of job loss.* Washington, DC: American Psychiatric Press.

Kernberg, O. (1967): Borderline personality organization. *Journal of the American Psychoanalytical Association, 15,* 641–685.

Kernberg, O. (1975). *Borderline conditions and pathological narcissism.* New York: Jason Aronson.

Kernberg, O. (1977). Normal psychology of the aging process, revisited II. Discussion. *Journal of Geriatric Psychiatry, 10,* 27–45.

Kernberg, O. (1980). *Internal world and external reality.* New York: Jason Aronson.

Kernberg, O. (1983, September). *Clinical aspects of narcissism.* Paper presented at Grand Rounds, Cornell University Medical Center, Westchester Division.

Kernberg, O. (1984). *Severe personality disorders.* New Haven, CT: Yale University Press.

Kernberg, O. (1985). *Clinical diagnosis and treatment of narcissistic personality disorder.* Paper presented at Swedish Association for Mental Health. Stockholm, Sweden.

Kernberg, O. (1989a). The narcissistic personality disorder and the differential diagnosis of antisocial behavior. *Psychiatric Clinics of North America, 12*(3), 553–570.

Kernberg, O. (Ed.). (1989b). Narcissistic Personality Disorder. *Psychiatric Clinics of North America, 12*(3).

Kernberg, O. (1990). Narcissistic personality disorder. In R. Michaels (Ed.), *Psychiatry* (chap. 18). Philadelphia: Lippincott-Raven.

Kernberg, O. (1992). *Aggression in personality disorders and perversions.* New Haven, CT: Yale University Press.

Kernberg, O. (1993a). Nature and agents of structural intrapsychic change. In M. J. Horowitz, O. Kernberg, & E. M. Weinshel (Eds.), *Psychic structure and psychic change—essays in honor of Robert S. Wallerstein* (pp. 327–344). Madison, CT: International Universities Press.

Kernberg, O. (1993b). Suicidal behavior in borderline patients. Diagnostic and psychotherapeutic considerations. *American Journal of Psychotherapy, 47,* 245–254.

Kernberg, O. (1998a). The psychotherapeutic management of psychopathic, narcissistic and paranoid transference. In T. Millon, E. Simonsen, M. Birket-Smith, & R. D. Davis, (Eds.), *Psychopathy: Antisocial, violent and criminal behavior* (pp. 372–392). New York: Guilford Press.

Kernberg, O. F. (1998b). Pathological narcissism and narcissistic personality disorder. Theoretical background and diagnostic classifications. In E. Ronningstam (Ed.), *Disorders of narcissism: Diagnostic, clinical and empirical implications* (pp. 29–51). Washington, DC: American Psychiatric Press.

Kernberg, O. (1998c). *Ideology, conflict, and leadership in groups and organiza-tions*. New Haven, CT: Yale University Press.

Kernberg, O. (1999). A severe sexual inhibition in the course of the psychoana-lytic treatment of a patient with a narcissistic personality disorder. *International Journal of Psychoanalysis, 80*, 899–908.

Kernberg, O. (2001). The suicidal risk in severe personality disorders: Dif-ferential diagnosis and treatment. *Journal of Personality Disorder, 15*(3), 195–208.

Kernberg, P. (1989). Narcissistic personality disorder in childhood. *Psychiatric Clinics of North America, 12*(3), 671–694.

Kernberg, P. (1998). Developmental aspects of normal and pathological narcis-sism. In E. Ronningstam (Ed.), *Disorders of narcissism: Diagnostic, clinical, and empirical implications* (pp. 103–120) Washington, DC: American Psy-chiatric Press.

Kernberg, P., F. Hajal, & L. Normandin. (1998). Narcissistic personality disorder in adolescent inpatients—a retrospective record review study of descrip-tive characteristics. In E. Ronningstam (Ed.), *Disorders of narcissism: Diag-nostic, clinical and empirical implications* (pp. 437–456). Washington, DC: American Psychiatric Press.

Kernis, M. H., D. P. Cornell, C.-R. Sun, A. Berry, & T. Harlow. (1993). There's more to self-esteem than whether it is high or low: The importance of stability of self-esteem. *Journal of Personality and Social Psychology, 65* (6), 1190–1204.

Kernis, M. H., B. D. Grannemann, & L. C. Barclay. (1989). Stability and level of self-esteem as predictors of anger arousal and hostility. *Journal of Personal-ity and Social Psychology, 56*(6), 1013–1022.

Kernis, M. H., & C.-R. Sun. (1994). Narcissism and reactions to interpersonal feedback. *Journal of Research on Personality, 28*, 4–13.

Kerr, N. J. (1985). Behavioral manifestations of misguided entitlement. *Perspec-tives in Psychiatric Care, 23*(1), 5–15.

Khantzian, E. J. (1979). Impulse problems in addictions: Cause and effect rela-tionships. In H. Wishnie (Ed.), *Working with the impulsive person* (pp. 97–112). New York: Plenum Press.

Khantzian, E. J. (1980). An ego-self theory of substance dependence: A contemporary psychoanalytic perspective. In D. J. Lettieri, M. Sayers, & H. W. Pearson (Eds.), *Theories on drug abuse* (NIDA Research Mono-graph No. 30; pp. 29–33). Rockville, MD: National Institute on Drug Abuse.

Khantzian, E. J. (1982). Psychological (structural) vulnerabilities and the spe-cific appeal to narcotics. *Annals of New York Academy of Science, 398*, 24–32.

Khantzian, E. J. (1985). The self-medication hypothesis of addictive disorders: Focus on heroin and cocaine dependence. *American Journal of Psychiatry, 142*, 1259–1264.

Klein, D. N., L. P. Riso, S. K. Donaldson, J. E. Schwartz, R. L. Anderson, P. C. Oiumette, H. Lizardi, & T. A. Aronson. (1995). Family study of early-onset dysthymia: Mood and personality disorders in relatives of outpatients with dysthymia and episodic major depressive and normal controls. *Archives of General Psychiatry. 52*, 487–496.

Klein, M. (1957). *Envy and gratitude*. New York: Basic Books.

Klein, M. (1958). On the development of mental functioning. *International Journal of Psychoanalysis, 39*, 84–90.

Kohut, H. (1966). Forms and transformations of narcissism. *American Journal of Psychotherapy, 14*, 243–271.

Kohut, H. (1968). The psychoanalytic treatment of narcissistic personality disorder. *Psychoanalytic Study of the Child, 23*, 86–113.

Kohut, H. (1971). *The analysis of the self*. New York: International Universities Press.

Kohut, H. (1972). Thoughts on narcissism and narcissistic rage. *The Psychoanalytic Study of the Child, 27*, 360–400.

Kohut, H. (1977). *The restoration of the self*. New York: International University Press.

Kohut, H., & E. S. Wolf (1978). The disorders of the self and their treatment: An outline. *International Journal of Psychoanalysis, 59*, 413–425.

Kriegman, G. (1983). Entitlement attitudes: Psychosocial and therapeutic implications. *The Journal of American Academy of Psychoanalysis, 11*(2), 265–281.

Krystal, H. (1998). Affect regulation and narcissism: Trauma, alexithymia and psychosomatic illness in narcissistic patients. In E. Ronningstam (Ed.), *Disorders of narcissism: Diagnostic, clinical and empirical implications* (pp. 299–325). Washington, DC: American Psychiatric Press.

Lansky, M. (1991). Shame and the problem of suicide: A family systems perspective. *British Journal of Psychotherapy, 7*(3), 230–242.

Lansky, M. (1997). Envy as a process. In M. R. Lansky & A. P. Morrison (Eds.), *The widening scope of shame* (pp. 327–338). Hillsdalem, NJ: Analytic Press.

Lester, D. (1998). The association of shame and guilt with suicidality. *Journal of Social Psychology, 138*, 535–536.

Levine, H. (1997). Men at work: Work, ego and identity in the analysis of adult men. In C. W. Socarides & S. Kramer (Eds.), *Work and its inhibitions: Psychoanalytic essays* (pp. 143–157). Madison CT: International Universities Press.

Lewin, R. (1992). On chronic suicidality. *Psychiatry, 55*, 16–21.

Lewis, H. B. (1971). *Shame and guilt in neurosis*. New York: International Universities Press.

Lewis, M. (1995). Embarrassment: The emotion of self-exposure and evaluation. In J. P. Tangney & K. W. Fischer (Eds.), *Self-conscious emotions: The psychology of shame, guilt, embarrassment and pride* (pp. 198–218). New York: Guilford Press.

Lichtenberg, J. D. (1987). An experiential approach to narcissistic and borderline patients. In J. S. Grothstein, M. F. Solomon, & J. A. Lang (Eds.), *The borderline patient—emerging concepts in diagnosis, psychodynamics and treatment* (Vol. 2, pp. 127–148). Hillsdale, NJ: Analytic Press.

Lindsay-Hartz, J. (1984). Contrasting experiences of shame and guilt. *American Behavioral Scientist, 27*, 689–704.

Livesley, W. J., D. N. Jackson, & M. Schroeder. (1992). Factorial structure of traits delineating personality disorders in clinical and general population samples. *Journal of Abnormal Psychology, 101*, 432–440.

Maccoby, M. (1981). *The leader, a new face for American management*. New York: Simon and Schuster.

Maccoby, M. (2000, January–February). The narcissistic leaders. The incredible pros, and the inevitable cons. *Harvard Business Review, 78*, 68–77.

Maccoby, M. (2002). *The productive narcissist*. New York: Reed Business Information.

Maffei, C., A. Fossati, V. Lingiardi, F. Madeddu, C. Borellini, & M. Petrachi. (1995). Personality maladjustment, defenses and psychopathological symptoms in non-clinical subjects. *Journal of Personality Disorders, 9*(4), 330–345.

Malin, A. (1990). Psychotherapy of the narcissistic personality disorders. In A. Tasman, S. M. Goldfinger, & C. A. Kaufman (Eds.), *American Psychiatric Press review of psychiatry* (Vol. 9, pp. 355–368). Washington, DC: American Psychiatric Press.

Malmquist, C. P. (1996). *Homocide: A psychiatric perspective*. Washington, DC: American Psychiatric Press.

Maltsberger, J. T. (1993). Confusion of the body, the self and others in suicidal states. In A. Leenaars (Ed.), *Suicidology: Essays in honor of Edwin S. Shneidman* (pp. 148–171). Northvale, NJ: Jason Aronson.

Maltsberger, J. T. (1996). Suicide danger: Clinical estimation and decision. *Suicide and Life Threatening Behavior, 18*(1), 47–54.

Maltsberger, J. T. (1997). Ecstatic suicide. *Archive of Suicide Research, 3*(4), 283–301.

Maltsberger, J. T. (1998). Pathological narcissism and self-regulatory processes in suicidal states. In E. Ronningstam (Ed.), *Disorders of narcissism: Diag-

nostic, clinical and empirical implications (pp. 327–344). Washington, DC: American Psychiatric Press.

Maltsberger, J. T., & D. H. Buie. (1973). Countertransference hate in the treatment of suicidal patients. *Archive of General Psychiatry, 30,* 625–633.

Masterson, J. F. (1981). *The narcissistic and borderline disorders.* New York: Brunner/Mazel.

Masterson, J. (1993). *The emerging self—a developmental, self, and object relations approach to the treatment of the closet narcissistic disorder of the self.* New York: Brunner/Mazel.

Mattia, J. I., & M. Zimmerman. (2001). Epidemiology. In W. J. Livesley (Ed.), *Handbook of personality disorders* (pp. 107–123). New York: Guilford Press.

McCann, J. T., & M. K. Biaggio. (1989). Narcissistic personality features and self-reported anger. *Psychological Reports, 64,* 55–58.

McDougall, J. (1985). *Theaters of the mind.* New York: Basic Books.

McGlashan, T., & R. Heinssen. (1989). Narcissistic, antisocial and non-comorbid subgroups of borderline patients. *Psychiatric Clinics of North America, 12* (3), 653–671.

Melville, A. D. (Trans.). (1986). *Ovid's Metamorphoses.* Oxford: Oxford University Press.

Mikulincer, M., O. Gilliath, V. Halevy, N. Avihou, S. Avidan, & N. Eshkoli. (2001). Attachment theory and reactions to others' needs: Evidence that activation of the sense of attachment security promotes empathic responses. *Journal of Personality and Social Psychology, 81*(6), 1205–1224.

Miles, C. (1977). Conditions predisposing to suicide: A review. *Journal of Nervous and Mental Disorders, 164,* 231–246.

Miller, C. M., D. G. Jacobs, & T. G. Gutheil. (1998). Talisman or taboo: The controversy of the suicide-prevention contract. *Harvard Review of Psychiatry, 6,* 78–87.

Miller, J. (1998). *On reflections.* London: National Gallery Publications.

Millon, T. (1981). *Disorders of personality DSM-III: Axis II.* New York: Wiley & Sons.

Millon, T. (1996). *Disorders of personality. DSM-IV and beyond* (2nd ed.). New York: Wiley-Interscience.

Millon, T. (1998). *DSM* narcissistic personality disorder. historical reflections and future directions. In E. F. Ronningstam (Ed.), *Disorders of narcissism: Diagnostic, clinical and empirical implications* (pp. 75–101). Washington, DC: American Psychiatric Press.

Millon, T., & R. Davis. (2000). *Personality disorders in modern life.* New York: John Wiley & Sons.

Millon, T., R. D. Davis, & C. Millon. (1996). *Millon Clinical Multiaxial Inventory—III manual.* Minnetonka, MN: National Computer Systems, Inc.

Modell, A. H. (1965). Right to a life: An aspect of superego development. *International Journal of Psychoanalysis, 45,* 323–331.

Modell, A. (1975). A narcissistic defense against affects and the illusion of self-sufficiency. *International Journal of Psychoanalysis, 56,* 275–282.

Modell, A. (1980). Affects and their non-communication. *International Journal of Psychoanalysis, 61*(2), 259–267.

Modell, A. (1991). Resistance to the exposure of the private self. *Contemporary Psychoanalysis, 27,* 731–737.

Morey, L. C. (1988). Personality disorders in *DSM-III* and *DSM-III-R*: An examination of convergence, coverage, and internal consistency. *American Journal of Psychiatry, 145,* 573–577.

Morey, L. C., & J. K. Jones. (1998). Empirical studies of the construct validity of narcissistic personality disorder. In E. Ronningstam (Ed.), *Disorders of narcissism: Diagnostic, clinical and empirical implications* (pp. 351–374). Washington, DC: American Psychiatric Press.

Morf, C. C., & F. Rhodewalt. (1993). Narcissism and self-evaluation maintenance: Explorations in object relations. *Personality and Social Psychology Bulletin, 19*(6), 668–676.

Morf, C. C., & F. Rhodewalt. (2001). Unraveling the paradoxes of narcissism: A dynamic self-regulatory processing model. *Psychological Inquiry, 12*(4), 177–196.

Morrison, A. P. (1983). Shame, the ideal self and narcissism. *Contemporary Psychoanalysis, 19,* 295–318.

Morrison, A. P. (1987). The eye turned inward: Shame and the self. In D. Nathanson (Ed.), *The many faces of shame.* (pp. 271–291). New York: Guilford Press.

Morrison, A. P. (1989). *Shame: The underside of narcissism.* Hillsdale, NJ: Analytic Press.

Moser-Ha, H. (2001). Working through envy. *International Journal of Psychoanalysis, 82,* 713–725.

Moses, R., & R. Moses-Hrushovski. (1990). Reflections on the sense of entitlement. *The Psychoanalytic Study of the Child, 45,* 61–78.

Murray, H. (1955). American Icarus. In A. Burton & R. Harris (Eds.), *Clinical studies in personality* (Vol. 2, pp. 615–641). New York: Harper.

Murray, J. M. (1964). Narcissism and the ego ideal. *Journal of the American Psychoanalytic Association, 12,* 477–511.

Näcke, P. (1899). Die sexuellen perversitäten in der irrenanstalt. *Psychiatriche en Neurologische Bladen, 3.*

Nemiah, J. C., & P. E. Sifneos. (1970). Affect and fantasy in patients with psychosomatic disorder. In O. W. Hill (Ed.), *Modern trends in psychosomatic medicine*, (Vol. 2, pp. 26–34). London: Butterworth.

Nestor, P. (2002). Mental disorders and violence: Personality dimensions and clinical features. *American Journal of Psychiatry, 159*, 1973–1978.

Orbach, I., M. Lotem-Peleg, & P. Kedem. (1995). Attitudes toward the body in suicidal, depressed, and normal adolescents. *Suicide and Life-Threatening Behavior, 25*, 211–221.

Ornstein P. (1998). Psychoanalysis of patients with primary self-disorder. In E. Ronningstam (Ed.), *Disorders of narcissism: Diagnostic, clinical, and empirical implications* (pp. 147–169). Washington, DC: American Psychiatric Press.

Papps, B. P., & R. E. O'Carroll. (1998). Extremes of self-esteem and narcissism and the experience and expression of anger and aggression. *Aggressive Behavior, 24*, 421–438.

Penney, L., & P. Spector. (2002). Narcissism and counterproductive behavior: Do bigger egos mean bigger problems? *International Journal of Selection and Assessment, 10(1–2)*, 126–134.

Perry, J. C. (1990). Personality disorders, suicide and self-destructive behavior. In D. Jacobs & H. Brown (Eds.), *Suicide: Understanding and responding* (pp. 157–169). Madison, CT: International Universities Press.

Perry, J. D. C., & J. C. Perry. (2004). Conflicts, defenses and the stability of narcissistic personality features. *Psychiatry: Interpersonal and Biological Processes, 27*, 310–330.

Pierce, C. M. (1978). Entitlement dysfunctions. *Australian and New Zealand Journal of Psychiatry, 12*, 215–219.

Plakun, E. M. (1987). Distinguishing narcissistic and borderline personality disorders using *DSM-III* criteria. *Comprehensive Psychiatry, 28*, 437–443.

Plakun, E. (1989). Narcissistic personality disorder. A validity study and comparison to borderline personality disorder. *Psychiatric Clinics of North America, 12(3)*, 603–620.

Plakun, E. M. (1990). Empirical overview of narcissistic personality disorder. In E. M. Plakun (Ed.), *New perspectives on narcissism* (pp. 101–149). Washington, DC: American Psychiatric Press.

Preston, S. D., & F. B. M. de Waal. (2002). Empathy: Its ultimate and proximate bases. *Behavioral and Brain Sciences, 25*, 1–72.

Pulver, S. E. (1999). Shame and guilt: A synthesis. *Psychoanalytic Inquiry 19(3)*, 388–406.

Rank, O. (1911). Ein Beitrag zum Narzissismus. *Jahrbuch fur Psychoanalytische und Psychopathologische Forschungen, 3*, 401–426.

Raskin, R. N., & C. S. Hall. (1979). A narcissistic personality inventory. *Psychological Reports, 45,* 590.

Raskin, R. N., & C. S. Hall. (1981). The narcissistic personality inventory: Alternative form reliability and further evidence of construct validity. *Journal of Personality Assessment, 45,* 159–162.

Raskin, R. N., J. Novacek, & R. Hogan. (1991). Narcissism, self-esteem, and defensive self-enhancement. *Journal of Personality, 59,* 19–38.

Raskin, R. N., & R. Shaw. (1988). Narcissism and the use of personal pronouns. *Journal of Personality, 52*(2), 393–404.

Raskin, R. N., & H. Terry. (1988). A principal-component analysis of the narcissistic personality inventory and further evidence of its construct validity. *Journal of Personality and Social Psychology, 54,* 890–902.

Reich, A. (1960). Pathological forms of self-esteem regulation. *The Psychoanalytic Study of the Child, 15,* 215–232.

Reich, J., W. Yates, & M. Nduaguba. (1989). Prevalence of *DSM-III* personality disorders in the community. *Social Psychiatry and Psychiatric Epidemiology, 24,* 12–16.

Reich, W. (1949). *Character analysis* (trans. TP Wolfe; 3rd ed.). New York: Orgone Institute Press. (Original work published 1933)

Reichman, J., & J. Flaherty. (1990). Gender differences in narcissistic styles. In E. M. Plakun (Ed.), *New perspective on narcissism* (pp. 71–100). Washington, DC: American Psychiatric Press.

Renik, O. (1993). Countertransference enactment and the psychoanalytic process. In M. J. Horowitz, O. Kernberg, & E. M. Weinshel (Eds.), *Psychic structure and psychic change. Essays in honor of Robert S. Wallerstein* (pp. 135–158). Madison, CT: International Universities Press.

Renik, O. (1998). The role of countertransference enactment in a successful clinical psychoanalysis. In S. Ellman & M. Moskowitz (Eds.), *Enactment—towards a new approach to the therapeutic relationship* (pp. 111–128). Northvale, NJ: Jason Aronson.

Rhodewalt, F., J. C. Madrian, & S. Cheney. (1998). Narcissism, self-knowledge organization, and emotional reactivity: The effect of daily experiences on self-esteem and affect. *Personality and Social Psychology Bulletin, 24*(1), 75–87.

Rhodewalt, F., & C. C. Morf. (1995). Self and interpersonal correlates of the narcissistic personality inventory: A review and new findings. *Journal of Research in Personality, 29,* 1–12.

Rhodewalt, F., & C. C. Morf. (1998). On self-aggrandizement and anger: A temporal analysis of narcissism and affective reactions to success and failure. *Journal of Personality and Social Psychology, 74,* 672–685.

Rhodewalt, F., & D. L. Sorrow. (2003). Interpersonal self-regulation: Lessons from the study of narcissism. In M. R. Leary & J. P. Tangney (Eds.), *Handbook in self and identity* (pp. 519–535). New York: Guilford Press.

Richman, J. A., J. A. Flaherty, & K. M. Rosendale. (1996). Perceived workplace harassment experiences and problem drinking among physicians: Broadening the stress/alienation paradigm. *Addiction, 91*(3), 391–403.

Rinsley, D. B. (1989). Notes on the developmental pathogenesis of narcissistic personality disorder. *Psychiatric Clinics of North America, 12*(3), 695–707.

Rizzuto, A-M., W.W. Meissner & D.H. Buie. (2004). *The dynamics of human aggression: Theoretical foundation and clinical application.* New York: Brunner-Routledge.

Roberts, A. (2003, June). Dancing to a new tune—a survey of the Nordic region. *The Economist (London), 367*(8328), 1–16.

Robins, R. W., & O. P. John. (1997). Effects of visual perspective and narcissism on self-perception: Is seeing believing? *Psychological Science, 8*(1), 37–42.

Ronningstam, E. (1992, May). *Pathological narcissism in a sample of anorexic subjects.* Presented at American Psychiatric Association 145th annual meeting, Washington, DC.

Ronningstam, E. (1996). Pathological narcissism and narcissistic personality disorder in Axis I disorders. *Harvard Review of Psychiatry, 3,* 326–340.

Ronningstam, E. (Ed.). (1998). *Disorders of narcissism: Diagnostic, clinical and empirical implications.* Washington, DC: American Psychiatric Press.

Ronningstam, E., & D. Anick. (2001). The interrupted career group—a preliminary report. *Harvard Review of Psychiatry, 9,* 234–243.

Ronningstam, E., & J. Gunderson. (1989). Descriptive studies on narcissistic personality disorder. *Psychiatric Clinics of North America, 12*(3), 585–601.

Ronningstam, E., & J. Gunderson. (1990). Identifying criteria for narcissistic personality disorder. *American Journal of Psychiatry, 147,* 918–922.

Ronningstam, E., & J. Gunderson. (1991). Differentiating borderline personality disorder from narcissistic personality disorder. *Journal of Personality Disorder, 5,* 225–232.

Ronningstam, E., & J. Gunderson. (1996). Narcissistic personality—a stable disorder or a state of mind? *Psychiatric Times, 13*(2), 35–36.

Ronningstam, E., J. Gunderson, & M. Lyons. (1995). Changes in pathological narcissism. *American Journal of Psychiatry, 152,* 253–257.

Ronningstam, E., & J. Maltsberger. (1998). Pathological narcissism and sudden suicide-related collapse. *Suicide and Life-Threatening Behavior, 28*(3), 261–271.

Rosenfeld, H. (1964). On the psychopathology of narcissism: A clinical approach. *International Journal of Psychoanalysis, 45,* 332–337.

Rosenfeld, H. (1971). A clinical approach to the psychoanalytic theory of the life and death instincts: An investigation into the aggressive aspects of narcissism. *International Journal of Psychoanalysis, 52,* 169–178.

Rosenfeld, H. (1987). *Impasses and interpretations.* London: Tavistock Publications.

Rosenstein, D., & H. A. Horowitz. (1996). Adolescent attachment and psychopathology. *Journal of Consulting and Clinical Psychology, 64*(2), 244–253.

Roskies, E, C. Louis-Guerin, & C. Fournier. (1993). Coping with job insecurity: How does personality make a difference? *Journal of Organizational Behavior, 14*(7), 617–630.

Rothstein, A. (1979). Oedipal conflicts in narcissistic personality disorders. *International Journal of Psychoanalysis, 60,* 189–199.

Rothstein, A. (1980). *The narcissistic pursuit for perfection.* New York: International Universities Press.

Rush, S. (2000). At one with death: Destructive narcissism. *Psychoanalytic Quarterly, 69,* 711–740.

Sadger, J. (1910). Ein Fall von multipler Perversion mit hysterischen Absenzen. *Jahrbuch fur Psychoanalytische und Psychopathologische Forschungen, 2,* 59–133.

Sandell, R. (1993). Envy and admiration. *International Journal of Psychoanalysis, 74,* 1213–1221.

Sandler, J., E. S. Person, & P. Fonagy (Eds.). (1991). *Freud's "On Narcissism: An Introduction."* New Haven, CT: Yale University Press.

Sato, T., K. Sakado, T. Uehara, S. Sato, K. Nishioka, & Y. Kasahara. (1997). Personality disorders using *DSM-III-R* in a Japanese clinical sample with major depression. *Acta Psychiatrica Scandinavica, 95,* 451–453.

Schmidtke, A., C. Loehr, B. Weinacker, S. Fekete, C. Haring, K. Michel, & B. Temesvary. (2000). Chronische Suizidalitaet: Epidemiologie [Chronic suicidal behavior: Epidemiology]. *Krankenhauspsychiatrie, 11*(Suppl. 2), 76–81.

Schore, A. (1991). Early superego development: The emergence of shame and narcissistic affect regulation in the practicing period. *Psychoanalysis and Contemporary Thought, 14,* 187–250.

Schore, A. (1994). *Affect regulation and the origin of the self.* Hillsdale, NJ: Lawrence Erlbaum.

Schore, A. (1998). Early shame experiences and infant brain development. In P. Gilbert & B. Andrews (Eds.), *Shame: Interpersonal behavior, psychopathology and culture* (pp. 57–77). New York: Oxford University Press.

Schwartz-Salant, N. (1982). *Narcissism and character transformation. The psychology of narcissistic character disorder.* Toronto: Inner City Books.

Semrud-Clikeman, M., & G. W. Hynd. (1990). Right hemispheric dysfunction in non-verbal learning disabilities: Social academic, and adaptive functioning in adults and children. *Psychological Bulletin, 107*(2), 196–209.

Simon, R. I. (2001). Distinguishing trauma-associated narcissistic symptoms from posttraumatic stress disorder: A diagnostic challenge. *Harvard Review of Psychiatry, 10*, 28–36.

Sixth Annual Meeting of the American Psychopathological Association. (1915). *Journal of Abnormal Psychology, 10*, 263–292.

Smalley, R. L., & J. E. Stake. (1996). Evaluation sources of ego-threatening feedback: Self-esteem and narcissistic effects. *Journal of Research in Personality, 30*, 483–495.

Smari, J., E. Arason, H. Hafsteinsson, & S. Ingimarsson. (1997). Unemployment, coping and psychological distress. *Scandinavian Journal of Psychology, 38*(2), 151–156.

Smith, G., A. Ruiz Sancho, & J. Gunderson. (2001). Intensive outpatient program for treatment of borderline personality disorder. *Psychiatric Services, 52*(4), 532–533.

Solomon, M. F. (1989). *Narissism and intimacy: Love and marriage in an age of confusion.* New York: Norton.

Sorotzkin, B. (1985). *The quest for perfectionism: Avoiding guilt or avoiding shame? Psychotherapy, 22*(3), 564–571.

Sours, J. A. (1974). The anorexia nervosa syndrome. *International Journal of Psychoanalysis, 55*, 567–576.

Spender, M. (1999). *From a high point: A life of Arshile Gorky.* Los Angeles: University of California Press.

Spielman, P. M. (1971). Envy and jealousy. An attempt at clarification. *The Psychoanalytic Quarterly, 40*, 59–82.

Stark, M. (1989). Work inhibition: A self-psychological perspective. *Contemporary Psychoanalysis, 25*(1), 135–158.

Steiger, H., L. Gauvin, S. Jabalpurwala. (1999). Hypersensitivity to social interactions in bulimic syndromes: Relationship to binge eating. *Journal of Consulting and Clinical Psychology, 67*, 765–775.

Steiger, H., S. Jabalpurwala, J. Champagne, & S. Stotland. (1997). A controlled study of trait narcissism in anorexia and bulimia nervosa. *International Journal of Eating Disorders, 22*(2), 173–178.

Steinberg, B. E., & R. J. Shaw. (1997). Bulimia as a disturbance of narcissism: Self-esteem and the capacity to self-soothe. *Addictive Behaviors, 22*(5), 699–710.

Stewart, H. (1990). Interpretation and other agents for psychic change. *International Review of Psychoanalysis, 17*, 61–69.

Stone, M. (1989). Long-term follow-up of narcissistic borderline patients. *Psychiatric Clinics of North America, 12*(3), 621–642.

Stone, M. (1993). *Abnormalities of personality: Within and beyond the realm of treatment.* New York: Norton.

Stone, M. (1998). Normal narcissism. An etiological and ethological perspective. In E. Ronningstam (Ed.), *Disorders of narcissism: Diagnostic, clinical, and empirical implications* (pp. 7–28). Washington, DC: American Psychiatric Press.

Stormberg, D, E. Ronningstam, J. Gunderson, & M. Tohen. (1998). Brief communication: Pathological narcissism in bipolar patients. *Journal of Personality Disorders, 12*(2), 179–185.

Tähkä, J. (1979). Alcoholism as a narcissistic disturbance. *Psychiatrica Fennica, 10*, 129–139.

Tangney, J. P. (1990). Assessing individual differences in proneness to shame and guilt: Development of the self-conscious affect and attribution inventory. *Journal of Personality and Social Psychology, 59*(1), 102–111.

Tangney, J. P. (1991). Moral affect: The good, the bad, the ugly. *Journal of Personality and Social Psychology, 61*, 598–607.

Tangney, J. P. (1995). Shame and guilt in interpersonal relations. In J. P. Tangney & K. W. Fischer (Eds.), *Self-conscious emotions: The psychology of shame, guilt, embarrassment and pride* (pp. 114–139). New York: Guilford Press.

Tangney, J. P., & K. W. Fischer (Eds.). (1995). *Self-conscious emotions: The psychology of shame, guilt, embarrassment and pride.* New York: Guilford Press.

Tangney, J. P., P. Wagner, C. Fletcher, & R. Gramzow. (1992). Shamed into anger? The relation of shame and guilt to anger and self-reported aggression. *Journal of Personality and Social Psychology, 62*(4), 669–675.

Tangney, J. P., P. Wagner, & R. Gramzow. (1992). Proneness to shame, proneness to guilt and psychopathology. *Journal of Abnormal Psychology, 101*(3), 469–478.

Tangney, J. P., P. Wagner, D. Hill-Barlow, D. E. Marschall, & R. Gramzow. (1996). Relation of shame and guilt to constructive versus destructive responses to anger across the lifespan. *Journal of Personality and Social Psychology, 70*(4), 797–809.

Tantam, D. (1988). Lifelong eccentricity and social isolation: Asperger's syndrome or schizoid personality disorder? *British Journal of Psychiatry, 153*, 783–791.

Tartakoff, H. (1966). The normal personality in our culture and the Nobel Prize complex. In R. M. Lowenstein, L. M. Newman, M. Schure, A. J. Solnit. (Eds.), *Psychoanalysis: A general psychology* (pp. 222–252). New York: International Universities Press.

Tatara, M. P. (1976). Cultural characteristics of taijin kyofu-sho (anthropo-phobia) and its psychotherapeutic treatment. *Hiroshima Forum for Psychology, 3*, 67–71.

Tatara, M. P. (1993). Patterns of narcissism in Japan. In J. Fiscalini & A. Grey (Eds.), *Narcissism and the interpersonal self* (pp. 223–237). New York: Columbia University Press.

Tedlow, J., V. Leslie, B. R. Keefe, J. Alpert, A. A. Nierenburg, J. F. Rosenbaum, & M. Fava. (1999). Axis I and Axis II disorder comorbidity in unipolar depression with anger attacks. *Journal of Affective Disorders, 52*, 217–223.

Torgersen, S., E. Kringlen, & V. Cramer. (2001). The prevalence of personality disorders in a community sample. *Archives of General Psychiatry, 58*(6), 590–596.

Torgersen, S., S. Lygren, P. A. Øien, I. Skre, S. Onstad, E. Edvardson, K. Tambs, & E. Kringeln. (2000). A twin study of personality disorders. *Comprehensive Psychiatry, 41*(6), 416–425.

Turley, B., G. Bates, J. Edwards, & H. Jackson. (1992). MCMI-II personality disorders in recent-onset bipolar disorders. *Journal of Clinical Psychology, 48*, 320–329.

Tyrer, P., J. Gunderson, M. Lyons, & M. Tohen. (1997). Special feature: Extent of comorbidity between mental state and personality disorders. *Journal of Personality Disorders, 11*(3), 242–259.

Ullman, L. (1976). *Förändringen* [The Change] Stockholm: Forum.

Vaglum, P. (1999). The narcissistic personality disorder and addiction. In J. Derksen, C. Maffei, & H. Groen (Eds.), *Treatment of personality disorders* (pp. 241–253). New York: Kluwer Academic/Plenum.

Vaillant, G. E. (1988). The alcohol-dependent and drug-dependent person. In A. M. Nicholi (Ed.), *The Harvard guide to modern psychiatry* (2nd ed., pp. 700–713). Cambridge, MA: Harvard University Press.

Vaillant, G. E., & C. P. Perry. (1980). Personality disorders. In H. Kaplan, A. Freedman, & G. Sadoch (Eds.), *The comprehensive textbook of psychiatry* (3rd ed., Vol. 1, pp. 958–986). Baltimore: Williams & Wilkins.

Vaknin, S. (1999). *Malignant self love—narcissism revisited.* Prague: Narcissus Publications.

Valera, J. (1934). *Genio y figura.* Madrid, Spain: Novelas y Cuenos. (Original work published 1897)

Van Dongen, C. (1996). Quality of life and self-esteem in working and non-working persons with mental illness. *Community Mental Health Journal, 32*(6), 535–548.

Viinamaeki, H, L. Niskanen, & K. Koskela. (1995). How do mental factors predict ability to cope with long-term unemployment? *Nordic Journal of Psychiatry, 49*(3), 183–189.

Volkan, V. D. (1979). The "glass bubble" of the narcissistic patient. In J. LeBoit & A. Capponi (Eds.), *Advances in the psychotherapy of the borderline patient* (pp. 405–431). New York: Jason Aronson.

Wälder, R. (1925). The psychoses: Their mechanisms and accessibility to influence. *International Journal of Psychoanalysis, 6,* 259–281.

Wallace, H.M., R.F., Baumeister. (2002). The performance of narcissists rice and falls with perceived opportunity for glory. *Journal of Personality and Social Psychology, 82*(5), 819–834.

Warren, M. P., & A. Capponi. (1995–1996). The place of culture in the etiology of the narcissistic personality disorder: Comparing the United States, Japan and Denmark. *International Journal of Communicative Psychoanalysis and Psychotherapy, 11,* 11–16.

Watson, P. J., & M. D. Biderman. (1993). Narcissistic personality inventory factors, splitting and self-consciousness. *Journal of personality assessment, 61*(1), 41–57.

Watson, P. J., S. O. Grisham, M. V. Trotter, & M. D. Biderman. (1984). Narcissism and empathy: Validity evidence for the narcissistic personality inventory. *Journal of Personality Assessment, 48*(3), 301–305.

Watson, P. J., R. D. Morris, & L. Miller. (1998). Narcissism and the self as a continuum: Correlations with assertiveness and hypercompetitiveness. *Imagination, Cognition and Personality, 17*(3), 249–259.

Weinberger J. L., & J. J. Muller. (1974). The American Icarus revisited: Phallic narcissism and boredom. *International Journal of Psychoanalysis, 55,* 581–586.

Westen, D., & L. Arkowitz-Westen. (1998). Limitations of Axis II in diagnosing personality pathology in clinical practice. *American Journal of Psychiatry, 155,* 1767–1771.

Wicker, F. W., G. C. Payne, & R. D. Morgan. (1983). Participant's description of guilt and shame. *Motivation and Emotions, 7,* 25–39.

Wilson, P. (Ed.). (1983). *Fear of being fat.* New York: Jason Aronson.

Wilson, S. (1985). The self-pity response: A reconsideration. In A. Goldberg (Ed.), *Progress in self psychology* (Vol. 1, pp. 178–190). New York: Guilford Press.

Winge, L. (1967). *The Narcissus theme in western European literature up to the early 19th century.* Stockholm: Glerups.

Wink, P. (1991). Two faces of narcissism. *Journal of Personality and Social Psychology, 61,* 590–597.

Winnicott, D. W. (1953). Transitional objects and transitional phenomena. *International Journal of Psychoanalysis, 34,* 1–9.

Winnicott, D. W. (1965). *The maturational process and the facilitating environment.* London: Hogart.

Wolff, S. (1995). *Loners: The life path of unusual children.* London: Rutledge.

World Health Organization. (1992). *International classification of diseases and related health problems* (10th rev. ed.). Geneva, Switzerland: Author.

Wurmser, L. (1974). Psychoanalytic considerations of the etiology of compulsive drug use. *Journal of American Psychoanalytic Association, 22*, 820–843.

Yates, W., A. I. Fulton, J. M. Gabel, & C. T. Brass. (1989). Personality risk factors for cocaine abuse. *American Journal of Public Health, 79*, 891–892.

Young, J. (1994). *Cognitive therapy for personality disorders: A schema-focused approach* (rev. ed). Sarasota, FL: Professional Resource Press.

Young, J. (1998). Schema-focused therapy for narcissistic patients. In E. Ronningstam (Ed.), *Disorders of narcissism: Diagnostic, clinical and empirical implications* (pp. 239–268). Washington, DC: American Psychiatric Press.

Zanarini, M. C. (2000). Childhood experiences associated with the development of borderline personality disorder. *Psychiatric Clinics of North America, 23*(1), 89–101.

Zanarini, M. C., J. G. Gunderson, F. R. Frankenburg, & D. L. Chauncey. (1990). Discriminating borderline personality disorder from other Axis I disorders. *American Journal of Psychiatry, 147*, 161–167.

Zelin, M. L., S. B. Bernstein, C. Hein, R. M. Jampel, P. G. Myerson, G. Adler, D. H. Buie, & A. M. Rizzuto. (1983). The sustaining fantasy questionnaire: Measurement of sustaining functions of fantasies in psychiatric inpatients. *Journal of Personality Assessment, 47*(4), 427–439.

Index

abused children, 60
accomplishment, 144–45, 187
achievement, 78–79, 146, 184, 185
addiction, 126–28
adolescence, 55, 59–62
Adolescence (Brockhurst), 5
adopted children, 60
affect dysregulation, 91–92, 111, 133
affect regulation
    impaired, 166–67
    and mentalization, 52–53
    neurobiological origins of, 51–52
    in pathological narcissism, 69, 70,
      72, 77, 83–92
    of shy narcissist, 103
    studies on, 20–21
    and suicide, 166–67
age, 64–66, 184
aggression, 8, 46, 69, 85–87, 89, 107,
    140
Akhtar, S., 10, 103, 116, 122
Akiskal, H.S., 122
alcohol, 127
Alexander, F., 185
alexithymia, 84, 132–33
Ali, Mohammed, 35
alter ego transference, 183
American Psychopathological Asso-
    ciation, 6
amorous type, 15
anger, 45–46, 69, 77, 85–88, 92

anorexia, 75, 128–29
antisocial behavior, 109–10, 114
antisocial personality disorder
    (ASPD), 25, 27, 78, 107, 109,
    110–11, 112, 114–15
anxiety, 54, 130–31, 144
apathy syndrome, 45
arrogance, 98, 146
arrogant type narcissistic personality
    disorder, 72, 75–100, 112
    affect regulation, 83–92
    anger and rage, 85–88
    arrogance, control, and hostility, 98
    empathy, 94–98
    entitlement, 93–94
    envy, 89–91
    exploitativeness, 99
    grandiosity, 77–78
    interpersonal commitment, 98–99
    interpersonal relationships, 92–100
    masochism and martyr roles,
      80–82
    mood and hypochondria, 91–92
    reactions to criticism, 82
    real or exaggerated achievements,
      78–79
    self-esteem regulation, 76–83
    shame, 88–89
art, 4–5, 136, 137
ASPD. *See* antisocial personality
    disorder

Asperger's syndrome, 132
attachment, 51, 54–55
Audiard, Jacques, 67
Austen Riggs Center, 25–26
autoeroticism, 4, 5
avoidance, 37
Axelrod, S., 135
Axis I disorders, 120–33
Axis II personality disorders, 113–20

Balint, E., 54
Balint, M., 54
barbiturates, 127
Barth, F.D., 90
Berglas, Steve, 42, 142–43
Bergman, Ingmar, 136–37
Berkowitz, D.A., 59
biosocial learning perspective, 21, 49
bipolar disorder, 74–75, 121–24,
    187
Blair, Bonnie, 35
Bleiberg, E., 55
body shape, 128
borderline personality disorder
    (BPD), 12–13, 27, 51, 78, 110,
    115–18, 121, 122
BPD. *See* borderline personality
    disorder
bulimia, 129
Bursten, Ben, 14
Bursten's typology, 14

Calderon de la Barca, Pedro, 4
career. *See* workplace
caregiver-child patterns, 51
Cephisus, 3
charlatan, 15
childhood
    affect regulation and mentaliza-
        tion, 52–53
    developmental copying, 55–56
    and family role, 59–62
    narcissism and attachment, 54–55
    narcissistic parenting, 56–59
    neurobiological origins of affect
        regulation, 51–52
    origins of narcissistic personality
        disorder, 49–50

classification, 54
closet narcissist, 10, 101
cocaine, 127, 128
cognitive perspective, 21–22
commitment, 98–99
compensatory narcissistic self-infla-
    tion, 6
compensatory type, 15
competition, 101
compromised entitlement, 34
control, 39, 74, 98
Cooper, A.M., 10, 98, 132, 141
corporate culture, 46
corrective disillusionment, 185–86
corrective life events, 185–86
corrosive life events, 187–88
countertransference, 183
craving type, 14
criticism, 82, 103, 117
cultural differences, 43–47

Dali, Salvador, 136, 137
death, 176
delusion, 131
depersonification, 56
depleted self, 12
depressive disorder, 121, 124–26,
    187
developmental copying, 55–56
Diagnostic Interview for Narcissism,
    26
disappointment, 184
disillusionment, 184, 185–86
disordered narcissism, 70
dissociation, 167–68
Dodes, L.M., 127
Don Juan of achievements, 9
drug abuse, 126–28
dynamic self-regulatory process, 23

eating disorders, 75, 128–29
Echo, 3, 4
Eco y Narciso (Calderon), 4
ego, 5, 6, 82, 140
ego-ideal, 32, 40
ego psychology, 18
elitist type, 15
Ellis, Havelock, 4, 5

emotions, 37–39, 47
empathy, 35–36, 47, 94–98, 103
employment. *See* workplace
empty depression, 124
entitlement, 47
  case vignette, 93–94
  in child, 50
  definition of, 93
  exaggerated, 34, 94
  and grandiosity, 34, 93
  in narcissistic personality disorder,
    76
  and naricissistic rage, 86
  normal, 32–34
envy, 37, 38–39, 47, 69, 70, 89–91,
  92, 95
ethics, 105
evil mother, 58
exaggerated entitlement, 34, 94
excitatory mechanisms, 51
exploitativeness, 99, 109, 115
extraordinary narcissism, 72

family role, 59–62
fanatic type, 15
Fenichel, O., 9
Fernando, J., 57
field dependency/independency, 44
Finland, 46
Fiscalini, J., 19–20
Fonagy, P., 52–53, 95, 167
Freud, Sigmund, 5, 6, 8, 31–32, 183

Gabbard, Glenn, 58, 144
Garber, B., 36
gender, 64
genetics, 50–51, 52
Genio y Figura (Valera), 4
genotype, 52
Gergely, G., 52–53, 95
Girl in the Mirror (Rockwell), 5
Glad, B., 108
glass bubble fantasy, 9
God complex, 7
Gorky, Arshile, 137
grandiosity
  definition of, 78
  with delusions, 131

and entitlement, 34, 93
fantasies of, 39–40, 76, 78, 83, 102,
  104, 115, 201
as feature of narcissistic personality
  disorder, 26–27, 77–78, 121
origin of, 50
and parenting, 51
repressed, 11–12
schizophrenia with, 131
in shy narcissist, 10, 45, 101, 102
of tyrants, 108–9
greed, 90
Gunderson, John, 26

Haneke, Michael, 67
healthy narcissism. *See* normal narcissism
histrionic personality disorder
  (HPD), 114, 118
Hitler, Adolph, 108
homosexuality, 5
Horowitz, M.J., 105
hostility, 80, 98, 99
HPD. *See* histrionic personality
  disorder
humiliation, 70, 80, 124, 148–57,
  187, 191
humility, 46
hyperthymia, 122, 123
hypochondria, 91–92, 103, 132–33
hypomania, 74, 122, 123

Icarus complex, 9
ICG. *See* Interrupted Career Group
idealizing, 183
inferiority, 5, 84, 191
inhibitory mechanisms, 51
instrumental narcissism, 57
interpersonal commitment, 98–99
interpersonal interactions, 138–39,
  183
interpersonal relationships, 23–24,
  35, 69, 73, 92–100, 184, 185,
  186
interpersonal relativeness, 103–4,
  186
Interrupted Career Group (ICG),
  149–57

Japan, 43, 44–45, 46
job loss, 148–49, 188–89
Jones, E., 7, 10
Jones, J.K., 98
Jurist, E.L., 52–53, 95

Kernberg, O., 11, 12, 18, 25, 85,
    106–7, 125, 127, 136, 160, 183,
    184
Kernberg, P., 56, 58, 60
Klein, M., 89, 162
Kohut, H., 11, 12, 18, 19, 25, 39, 86,
    135, 183, 184
Kriegman, G., 34
Krystal, H., 167

Lansky, M., 168–69
leadership, 136
learning disabilities, 131–32
libido, 5, 54
life events, 184
    case vignettes, 188–96
    corrective, 185–86
    corrosive, 187–88
Liriope, 3

Maccoby, M., 136
malicious envy, 90–91
malignant narcissism, 18, 106–9, 114
Malmquist, C.P., 107
Maltsberger, J.T., 106, 162, 170
manipulative type, 14
martyr role, 80–82
masochism, 80–82, 101
Masterson, J., 10
McLean Hospital, 25, 26
MCMI. See Millon Clinical Multiaxial
    Inventory
mentalization, 36, 52–53
middle age, 65, 184
Millon, Theodore, 14, 21
Millon Clinical Multiaxial Inventory
    (MCMI), 16, 21, 28
Millon's typology, 14–16
mirroring, 5, 52, 183
Modell, A., 9–10, 56, 84
mood, 76, 91–92, 123, 175
morality, 105–6

Morey, L.C., 98
Morrison, A.P., 11, 20
motherhood, 57–58
movies, 66–67, 136–37
murder, 107
Murray, H., 9

Näcke, Paul, 5
narcissistic affect dysregulation, 4
narcissistic behavior disorder, 11
narcissistic disorder. See narcissistic
    personality disorder
narcissistic disturbance, 70
narcissistic libidinal type, 8
narcissistic-masochistic character,
    10–11
narcissistic object choice, 32
narcissistic parenting, 56–59, 61
narcissistic personalities, 7–11, 66–67
narcissistic personality disorder
    (NPD), 11–16
    and affect regulation, 69, 70, 72,
        77, 83–92, 103
    age differences in, 64–66, 184
    versus antisocial personality disor-
        der and psychopathy, 114–15
    and anxiety disorders, 130–31
    arrogant, 72, 75–100, 112
    and attachment, 54–55
    Austen Riggs and McLean Hospi-
        tal studies, 25–26
    and bipolar disorder, 121–24
    and borderline personality disor-
        der, 12–13, 115–18
    changes in, 181–96
    cognitive perspective, 21–22
    criteria for long-term stability, 111
    and cultural differences, 43–44
    definitions of, 70
    and depressive disorder, 124–26
    diagnosis of, 62–63
    DSM-IV criteria, 26–28, 70,
        75–76, 82, 113–14, 201
    and eating disorders, 128–29
    ego psychological/object relations
        approach, 18
    exclusion criteria for, 110–11
    and gender, 64

heritability of, 50–51, 182
identifying, 69–112
interface with Axis I disorders, 120–33
interface with Axis II personality disorders, 113–20
interpersonal approach, 19–20
and interpersonal relationships, 69, 73, 92–100
origins of, 49–62
prevalence of, 62–63
psychoanalytic perspective, 16–21
psychopathic, 72, 105–10, 112
research on, 24–29
scope of, 62–66
and self-esteem regulation, 6, 72, 74–75, 76–83, 101–2, 104, 182, 186
self psychological approach, 19
shy, 72, 100–105, 112
social psychological perspective, 22–24
and substance-use disorders, 126–28
and suicide, 159–60
treatment of, 182–84
typologies, 14–16
Narcissistic Personality Inventory, 22, 28–29
narcissistic rage, 86, 87, 169–70, 194
narcissistic scientist, 7
narcissistic traits, 70, 71, 74–75, 117
Narcissus (Caravaggio), 4
Narcissus myth, 3–4, 136
neurobiological patterns, 51
Nobel Prize complex, 8–9
nonentitlement, 34
nonverbal learning disorder, 131–32
normal narcissism, 31–39, 72
    and control, power, and rage, 39
    definition of, 31
    and empathy, 35–36
    versus pathological narcissism, 69
    self-conscious emotions, 37–39
    self-preservation and entitlement, 32–34
    self-reference, 34–35
normal narcissistic type, 15

NPD. See narcissistic personality disorder

object relations, 18, 32
obsessive-compulsive personality disorder (OCD), 114, 118–19
OCD. See obsessive-compulsive personality disorder
Oedipal strivings, 57
old age, 65
opiates, 127
Ovid, 3

pain, 177–79
panic disorders, 130–31
paranoid personality disorder, 114, 119–20
paranoid psychosis, 131
paranoid type, 14
parenting, 50, 51, 52–53, 56–61
pathological narcissism. See narcissistic personality disorder
Penney, L., 140
perfectionism, 39–40, 105, 118–19
performance-related shame, 144–45
Perry, C.J., 159
personal development, 184
personality disorders, 54, 159, 187
    See also narcissistic personality disorder; specific personality disorders
phallic-narcissistic character, 8, 14, 21
phenotype, 52
Piano Teacher, The (movie), 67
Plakun, Erik, 25, 29
political leadership, 108
posttraumatic stress disorder (PTSD), 130, 187
power, 39
private self, 9–10, 56
psychedelic drugs, 127
Psychiatric Clinics of North America, 29
psychiatry, 5–7
psychoanalysis, 5–7, 16–21, 183
psychopathy, 72, 105–10, 112, 114–15
psychosis, 6, 11, 131

psychosomatic illness, 91, 132
PTSD. *See* posttraumatic stress
    disorder
publications, 29

rage, 85–88
    and addiction, 127
    and affect regulation, 70, 84
    "catastrophic reaction," 39
    in corrosive life events, 187
    entitled, 117
    and envy, 90
    inappropriate, 46
    narcissistic, 86, 87, 169–70, 194
    and suicide, 168–70
Read My Lips (movie), 67
recalling, 175
reflection, 5
Reich, Anne, 6
Reich, W., 8
restricted entitlement, 34
Rhodewalt, F., 23–24, 76
Rinsley, D.B., 56
Rorschach method, 29
Rosenfeld, H., 54, 89
Rothstein, A., 57

Saddam Hussein, 108
Sadger, J., 4, 5
sadism, 106, 107
Scandinavia, 43, 46
schizoid personality disorder, 114,
    120, 132
schizophrenia, 11, 131
Schore, A., 51, 53, 77, 167
self-aggrandizement, 78–79
self-cohesion, 19
self-conscious emotions, 37–39, 47
self-depreciation, 37
self-destructive behavior, 110, 117
self-esteem
    dysregulation, 34, 77, 83, 90, 101,
        111
    and eating disorders, 128–29
    and entitlement, 34
    healthy, 31
    instability, 76
    and narcissistic-masochistic char-
        acter, 10–11

in narcissistic personality disorder,
    70, 72, 74–75, 76–83, 101–2,
    121, 182, 186
    parental, 59
    and parenting, 51
    positive, 39
    regulation, 6, 17, 23, 28, 34, 72,
        74–75, 76–83, 85, 101–2, 104,
        176–79, 182, 186
    and shame, 77, 129
    and success, 40
    and suicide, 176–79
    threats to, 27, 78
self-pity, 80
self-preservation, 32, 86
self-reference, 34–35, 83
self-regard, 32
self-righteousness, 80
self-soother mood, 22
sexual perversion, 5, 106–7
shame
    and affect dysregulation, 92
    and affect regulation, 69, 70
    and anger, 88–89
    in corrosive life events, 187
    cultural tolerance of, 45–46
    and interpersonal relationships,
        89, 95
    Morrison on, 11, 124
    and narcissism, 88, 101
    performance-related, 144–45
    as self-conscious emotion, 37–38,
        47
    and self-esteem, 77, 129
    studies on, 20–21
    and suicide, 168–70
Shapiro, E.R., 59
Shapiro, R.L., 59
shy narcissistic personality, 10, 45–46,
    72, 100–105, 112
sliding meanings, 17, 105
social psychological perspective,
    22–24
somatization, 132–33
special self mood, 22
Spector, P., 140
stage fright, 141, 144
Stalin, Josef, 108
Stone, M., 32, 107

sublimation of narcissism, 6
substance-use disorders, 126–28
success, 39–43
success syndrome, 42
suicide and suicidality, 159–80
    in absence of depression, 125,
        162–66
    assessment and treatment of,
        170–76
    case vignettes, 87–88, 163–65,
        173–75, 177–79, 192
    chronic, 176–80
    and dissociation, 167–68
    facets of narcissistic patient,
        166–70
    and impaired affect regulation,
        166–67
    in malignant narcissism, 106
    narcissistic meaning of, 161–62
    and self-esteem regulation,
        176–79
    and shame and rage, 168–70
superego, 18, 70, 73, 105–6, 114
superiority, 75, 83, 88, 104

taijin kyofu sho, 44
Tangney, J.P., 88–89
TANS. See trauma-associated narcis-
    sistic symptoms
Target, M., 52–53, 95
Tartakoff, H., 8
Tatara, M., 44
therapeutic interventions, 183–84
tragic man, 11
transference, 6, 19, 183

trauma-associated narcissistic symp-
    toms (TANS), 70, 130, 196
Twemlow, S.W., 58
twin studies, 50, 182
tyranny, 108–9

unemployment, 148–49
uniqueness, 78, 83, 104
unprincipled type, 15

Vaglum, P., 128
Valera, Juan, 4
vanity, 4
Venus portraits, 4
violence, 109–10
Volkan, V.D., 9
vulnerable child mood, 22

Wälder, R., 7
weight, 75, 128
Western cultures, 43
workplace, 135–57
    career interruptions, 148–57, 187
    corrective experiences, 146–48
    counterproductive work behavior,
        140–41
    inhibitions, 141–45
    interpersonal interactions in,
        138–39
    Interrupted Career Group (ICG),
        149–57
    necessary niche in, 139–40
writer's block, 141

Zinner, J., 59